Breast Fitness

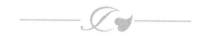

Breast Fitness

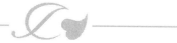

An Optimal Exercise and Health Plan
for Reducing Your Risk of Breast Cancer

ANNE MCTIERNAN, M.D., PH.D.

JULIE GRALOW, M.D.

LISA TALBOTT

St. Martin's Press ⚍ New York

www.stmartins.com

Design by Donna Sinisgalli

ISBN 0-312-25312-5

First Edition: October 2000

10   9   8   7   6   5   4   3   2   1

This book is dedicated

to the women who are confronting breast cancer.

They are our teachers in our quest

to learn how to fight this disease,

from prevention to cure.

A Note to Readers

This book is for informational purposes only. Readers are advised to consult a trained medical professional before acting on any of the information in this book. The fact that another book or an organization is listed in this book as a potential source of information does not mean that the authors or publisher endorses any of the information it may provide or recommendations it may make.

Research about breast cancer is ongoing. Although we have endeavored to use the most up-to-date information, there is no guarantee that what we know about this complex subject won't change with time.

Contents

Acknowledgments

We are grateful to many people who have provided inspiration, assistance, and guidance throughout the production of this book. First, we thank our families for their love and support, especially Cassie, Corina, Rachel, Hugh, and Martin.

Our agent, Nancy Crossman, has held our figurative hands throughout the whole process and has served as a deep source of guidance for us. We thank her for her faith in us and for showing us the way. We thank the many individuals at St. Martin's Press who made this book possible, especially our editor, Jennifer Weis, for her insights and wisdom. We also thank Joanna Jacobs for her valuable assistance.

We thank David Ehlert for artwork, Clayton Hibbert for graph design, Paul Zakar for photography, and Mari O'Neill, P.T., for modeling. We thank the breast cancer survivors who shared their thoughts and feelings with us and with you. Their bravery in facing their disease has inspired us. In particular we acknowledge Becky Galentine, Julie Macke, Beth Rowan, Kathy Uranich, and Marcia Vickery. We thank our Team Survivor colleagues, including Mary Berg, Denise Bowls, Julia Cañas, Carla Felsted, Nina Fogg, Michelle Kunzwiler, Monica Packard, Janet Parker, Marisa Perdomo, Beverly Sigler, Dana Sigley, and Karen Van Kirk, who have been great leaders in the growth of the Team Survivor wellness concept. The people who volunteer and support Team Survivor programs have all contributed in various ways to this book by their incredible dedication to the cause. We thank Sally Edwards, Maggie Sullivan, and the staff at the Danskin Women's Triathlon Series for their contribution to the empowerment of women cancer survivors through their Danskin Team Survivor programs.

We thank the women who have served as participants in our research studies at the Fred Hutchinson Cancer Research Center and the University of Washington. They are all pioneers in discovering how the biology of exercise and of cancer intersects. We thank the kind benefactors who have helped to support our exercise studies at the Fred Hutchinson Cancer Research Center and our exercise programs at Team Survivor and Cancer Lifeline.

We thank our colleagues at Fred Hutchinson Cancer Reseach Center, the University of Washington, and Cancer Lifeline. We appreciate the efforts of the researchers who work with us in exercise and breast cancer, including: Deborah Bowen, Ph.D., Melinda Irwin, Ph.D., John Potter, M.D., Ph.D., Rebecca Rudolph, M.D., M.P.H., Anna Schwartz, A.R.N.P., Ph.D., Robert Schwartz, M.D., Cornelia Ulrich, Ph.D., Mark Wener, M.D., Brent Wood, M.D., and Yutaka Yasui, Ph.D. Without the dedication and perseverence of our research staff, the studies would not get done. We appreciate the many efforts and dedication of: Marcelle Aquino, Erin Aykard, Jim Brockmeier, Patricia Cherney, Rob Hastings, M.Ed., Claudia Kumai, P.A., Kristin LaCroix, M.P.H., Kim Mabee, Angie Morgan, M.S., Lynda McVarish, M.Sc., Heather Nakamura, M.P.E., M.S., R.D., Liza Noonan, M.S., Judy Schramm R.N., Shelley Slate, and Danielle Yancey. We thank Barbara Frederick and the staff at Cancer Lifeline for their support and knowing voice when articulating the needs of women living with cancer. We thank Dr. Robert Livingston, M.D., for his mentorship in breast cancer treatment and research. There are many others, too numerous to list, who have helped in our efforts. We thank you also.

We are grateful to the many people who generously read and critiqued the book for their time and valuable input: Vicki Boehman, Amy Buckalter, EllenAnn Chidixx, Sally Edwards, Meg Honan, P.T., Melinda Irwin, Ph.D., Angela Lim, Karen Lindsley, M.D., Heather Nakamura, M.P.E., M.S., R.D., Paula Oliver, M.D., Marisa Perdomo, P.T., Carolyn Price, Lynne Sitton, Rändi Sundby, P.T., Toni Talbott, Kathe Wallace, P.T., and Colleen Zakar, R.N.

Breast Fitness

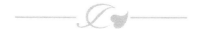

1

Introduction

You are your own primary health care provider. No health professional can provide the same amount of individual attention, focus, and energy that you can provide for your own health care. Women make the majority of health decisions for themselves and their families. In doing this, they are now arming themselves with more and better information about how best to promote health, avoid disease, and maintain a sense of well-being.

Breast cancer is at the top of most women's minds. They want to know what they can do to prevent breast cancer from happening to them or their loved ones. Women who are living with breast cancer want to know what they can do to prevent a recurrence of the disease, enhance their quality of life, and improve their chances of surviving.

Scientists now believe that lifestyle changes can make a profound impact on a woman's risk of developing breast cancer. Some of the things that may cause breast cancer can also be related to chance of long-term survival for women who already have the disease. We know that compared with thin women, women who are overweight or obese have almost *twice the risk* of getting breast cancer after menopause. Women of any age with breast cancer who are overweight or obese have *twice the risk* of not surviving for five or ten years after diagnosis, compared with lighter women. Exercise is an excellent way to fight excess weight and control obesity. It makes sense, then, that if exercise protects women from getting breast cancer, it might also reduce recurrence for women who have had breast cancer. After breast cancer surgery and treatment, exercise helps women rehabilitate themselves both physically and emotionally.

We have worked with hundreds of women, with and without breast cancer, who have made the commitment to their own health by making exercise a regular part of their lives. We wrote this book so that we could tell you their stories and so that we could share with you what we have learned about the role of exercise in fighting breast cancer. We give you up-to-date medical and scientific information from recent research. We teach you what kind of exercises will help you to improve your health. We provide step-by-step instructions on how to start and stick with an exercise program and how to avoid injuries. Throughout the book, we introduce you to women who have already taken these steps to improve their lives. You'll be inspired with the stories of cancer survivors who have made exercise a top priority for their own health and who have found new joys in working out with other survivors. Their strength and courage will convince you that you too can reach your goals of increasing fitness and strength and reducing your risk of diseases such as breast cancer.

All a woman can do is to work with what she has the power over— her own life and her own body. There is no greater sense of peace than to know in your heart and soul that you are living the life you choose and not waiting for choices to be made for you.

2

Breast Cancer Statistics
and Risk Factors

As we enter the new millennium, a new breast cancer will be diagnosed every three minutes in the United States, and a woman will die from breast cancer every twelve minutes. We believe that breast cancer is largely preventable and treatable. We also believe that more lives are being saved, and even more can be saved, using knowledge and technology that are available today. New ways are being discovered of detecting early breast cancer, treating all stages of the disease, and preventing cancers from developing in the first place. From this knowledge and experience, we have faith that our work in fighting cancer will have great results and will save lives. In this chapter, we give you some basic information on the biology of breast cancer. We present the statistics—the number of women expected to develop breast cancer each year and the number expected to die from this disease. We then outline the current knowledge on what increases or decreases risk for breast cancer.

What Is Breast Cancer?

Breast cancer is a malignant tumor that has developed from the cells of the breasts. The main components of the female breast are lobules (milk-producing glands), ducts (milk passages that connect the lobules and the nipple), and stroma (fatty tissue and ligaments surrounding the ducts and lobules, blood vessels, and lymphatic vessels). If breast cancer always stayed confined to the breast, it would not be life-threatening. The problem is that the breast cancer cells migrate into the nearby lymph vessels and blood vessels and travel to other parts of the body where they can multiply, grow, and interfere with critical organ functioning. This is why it is so important to detect breast cancer at a very early stage, before it has had the chance to spread elsewhere in the body.

✑ Breast Cancer Statistics

Breast cancer is the most common life-threatening cancer in women in the United States: A woman who lives into her eighties has a one in nine chance of developing breast cancer. In 1960, a woman's lifetime chance of getting breast cancer was only one in fourteen. Luckily, this increase in the chance of developing breast cancer has leveled off in the 1990s. In 1999, more than 180,000 American women developed breast cancer, and another 40,000 women were diagnosed with in situ, or preinvasive, breast cancer. Approximately three-fourths of women with breast cancer in the United States are over age fifty, and half of all breast cancers occur in women sixty-five years old and older. These statistics are complied yearly by the American Cancer Society. See Appendix B for information on how to reach them.

Table 2.1. Chance of Women Developing Breast Cancer
by Certain Ages

AGE	CHANCE OF DEVELOPING BREAST CANCER
By age 40	1 in 200
By age 50	1 in 50
By age 60	1 in 25
Birth to death	1 in 8

✑ Breast Cancer Survival

Although one in nine women in the United States will develop breast cancer, only one in thirty will die from this disease. The American Cancer Society estimated that 43,300 women in the United States died from breast cancer in 1999. Breast cancer is the second leading cause of cancer death in women, after lung cancer. It is the leading cause of cancer death among women age forty to fifty-five years. Although there is some fluctuation in the numbers, it looks as if the death rate from breast cancer is falling. In the early 1990s, the death rate for breast cancer dropped approximately 5 percent. This may be due to earlier detection, better treatment, or both.

The five-year survival rate for localized breast cancer has increased from 72 percent in the 1940s to 97 percent today. If the cancer has spread regionally (to the lymph nodes), the five-year survival rate is 77 percent. For women with distant metastases, this rate is 22 percent. As many as 69 percent of all women diagnosed with breast cancer survive ten years, and fifty-seven percent survive fifteen years. Research suggests that the death rate from breast cancer could decrease by 30 percent if all women followed screening mammography guidelines. That translates into almost 12,000 lives saved each year! Early detection of breast cancer gives a woman her best chance for survival.

What Causes Breast Cancer?

Although we know some of the risk factors that increase a woman's chances of developing breast cancer, we do not yet understand what causes most breast cancers. Researchers are making great progress in understanding how certain changes in DNA can cause normal cells to become cancerous. DNA is the chemical that carries the instructions for nearly everything our cells do. Some genes (parts of DNA) contain instructions for controlling when our cells grow, divide, and die. We know that cancer can be caused by DNA mutations (changes) that "turn on" oncogenes—cancer-related genes that promote cell division—or "turn off" tumor suppressor genes. An error in DNA that results in the activation of an oncogene is like stepping down on the accelerator of a car—it speeds up cell growth and division. Tumor suppressor genes slow down cell division or cause cells to die at the right time. An error in DNA that results in the disabling of a tumor suppressor gene is like letting up on the brakes of a car—it speeds up cell growth and division.

Certain inherited DNA changes can cause some cancers to occur very frequently and are responsible for cancers that run in some families.

Most DNA mutations related to breast cancer occur during a woman's life rather than having been inherited from her parents or distant ancestors. These are the DNA changes that are most likely due to a woman's environment (such as from radiation or chemicals) or lifestyle. So far, studies have not been able to identify any particular chemical in the environment or in our diets that is likely to cause these mutations.

Breast Cancer Risk Factors

A risk factor is anything that increases your chance of getting a disease. Different cancers have different risk factors. Having one risk factor, or even several, does not necessarily mean that you will develop the disease. Some women with one or more breast cancer risk factors never develop the disease, while many breast cancer patients have no obvious risk factors. Even when a patient has a risk factor, there is no way to prove that it caused her breast cancer.

There are different kinds of risk factors. Some, like a person's age, family history, and gender, can't be changed. Others are linked to cancer-causing factors in the environment. Still others are related to personal choices, such as lack of exercise, inadequate diet, and drinking alcohol.

Some factors influence risk more than others. For example, advancing age, personal history of breast cancer, and family history of breast cancer are risk factors that could increase a woman's risk to above that of the average woman. A woman's risk for developing breast cancer can change over time. A change in risk could be caused by increasing age or a new breast biopsy result. A young woman may not think about having a genetic risk for breast cancer if no one in her family has had the disease. If her mother or sister develops breast cancer, then all of a sudden the woman is now at increased risk by virtue of having a new diagnosis of breast cancer in the family.

A Personal History of Breast Cancer

A woman with breast cancer in one breast has a three- to fourfold increased risk of developing a new cancer in the other breast compared with women who have never had breast cancer. There are some women who are most likely to get a second cancer, including women who are younger when they got their first cancer and women with a strong family history of breast cancer. Treatment with tamoxifen seems to reduce the chance of developing a second breast cancer by about half.

Gender and Age

The two strongest risk factors for developing breast cancer are being a woman and getting older. Although men can develop this disease, male breast cancer occurs very rarely. Women are at least one hundred times more likely to get breast cancer compared with men. In the United States, the average age at breast cancer diagnosis is sixty-two, and three-quarters of all breast cancers occur in women over age fifty. Women age twenty to twenty-nine account for less than one half of 1 percent of breast cancer cases.

Figure 2.1. Female breast cancer incidence and death rates, by age and race, 1992–1996

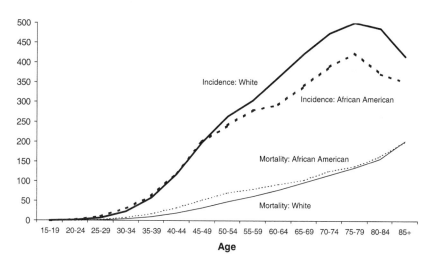

Source: American Cancer Society's Cancer Facts and Figures—1999. Reprinted with permission. Data sources: U.S. Mortality 1973–1996, National Center for Health Statistics, Centers for Disease Control and Prevention 1999; SEER Incidence 1973–1996, Surveillance, Epidemiology, and End Results Program, Division of Cancer Control and Population Sciences, National Cancer Institute. Graph design by Clayton Hibbert.

✍ Race and Ethnicity

Caucasian women have the highest risk of getting breast cancer in this country. However, the risk of breast cancer is considerable in other racial and ethnic groups. Of particular concern is the increasing rate of breast cancer occurrence in African-American women, particularly younger women. In fact, in women under age fifty, the risk for African-American women is greater than for Caucasian women. American women who are of Asian, Native American, or Hispanic origin have lower rates of breast cancer compared with Caucasian women. However, their risk is still considerable, and it is higher than the rates of breast cancer in women of similar race or ethnic backgrounds in other countries.

Even though women of color in America are at considerable risk of getting breast cancer, they are not getting screened for this disease at the same rate as white women. The reasons for this are not clear but might include access to, or acceptability of, screening mammograms and clinical breast exams. Or it may be that the cost of a mammogram is prohibitive to women with lower incomes or who are uninsured. The unfortunate

Figure 2.2. Female breast cancer incidence rates by race and ethnicity, 1973–1996

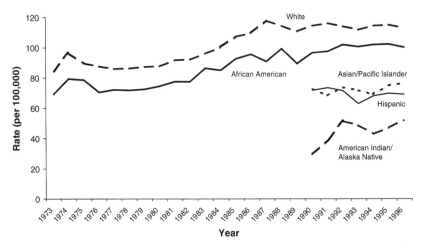

Source: American Cancer Society's Cancer Facts and Figures—1999. Reprinted with permission. Rates are age adjusted to the 1970 U.S. standard population. American Cancer Society, Surveillance Research, 1999. Data source: NCI Surveillance, Epidemiology, and End Results Program, 1999. Graph design by Clayton Hibbert.

result of this lack of screening is that if a woman of color gets breast cancer in this country, she is more likely to have advanced disease and more likely to die of breast cancer, compared with a white woman who gets breast cancer. The prevention of new and recurrent breast cancer is therefore a vitally important issue for *all* American women.

Family History and Genetics

As many as eight in ten women with breast cancer are the first ones in their families to develop the disease; that is, they have no family history of breast cancer. Nevertheless, your risk of developing breast cancer is higher than average if you have female relatives who have had the disease. This risk increases when family members develop breast cancer at a younger age (less than fifty), develop cancer in both breasts, or are closely related (mother, sisters). The inherited genes can be passed down either from your mother's or your father's side of the family.

The "Breast Cancer" Genes

About 5 to 10 percent of all breast cancers are due to inherited genes. Two breast cancer susceptibility genes, BRCA1 and BRCA2, have been identified so far. Women who inherit a mutated form of one of these genes have a high risk of developing breast and ovarian cancer. In families with inherited forms of breast cancer, there are typically more than two first-degree relatives (mother, daughter, sister) with breast or ovarian cancer, and breast cancer occurs at young age (forties, thirties, or even twenties).

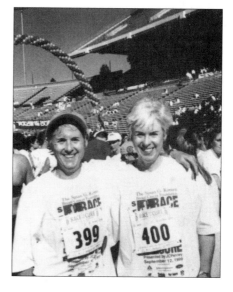

Nina Fogg (left) with twin sister, Carolyn

Normally, the BRCA1 and BRCA2 genes help to prevent cancer by making proteins that keep cells from growing abnormally. If a woman has inherited a mutated gene from either parent, however, this cancer-preventing protein is less effective, and the chances of developing cancer increase.

There is a 50 percent chance that the abnormal copy of a BRCA1 or BRCA2 gene carried by a parent will be passed on to a child. Women who inherit an abnormal form of BRCA1 or BRCA2 are highly susceptible to breast and ovarian cancers. Women of Ashkenazi Jewish descent, particularly those with a family history of breast or ovarian cancer, have a higher-than-average risk of carrying a particular abnormal form of the BRCA1 or BRCA2 gene. About 50 to 60 percent of women with BRCA1 or BRCA2 mutations will develop breast cancer by the age of seventy. Women with these mutations also have an increased risk for developing ovarian cancer. Men and women with a BRCA1 mutation have a slightly higher lifetime risk of developing colon cancer, and men have increased risk for prostate cancer.

Mutations of the p53 tumor suppressor gene can also increase a woman's risk of developing breast cancer, as well as leukemias, sarcomas, and brain tumors. The Li-Fraumeni syndrome, an inherited mutation in the p53 gene, is a rare cause of breast cancer.

A genetic test uses a blood sample to analyze DNA from a person to see if she has inherited a mutated BRCA1 or BRCA2. Testing the p53 gene is not part of usual breast cancer genetic testing but may be done if the family history raises the possibility of Li-Fraumeni syndrome. If a mutated gene is found, the woman and her health care team can use this information to make decisions about breast cancer prevention strategies and the frequency of breast cancer screening tests. Some women at very high risk of developing breast cancer may choose to have a prophylactic mastectomy (surgery to remove the breasts before cancer develops). Physicians may also recommend removal of the ovaries after childbearing or menopause, due to the increased risk of ovarian cancer in BRCA1 and BRCA2 gene mutation carriers.

Screening the general population for these breast cancer genes is unlikely to be beneficial. A woman who tests negative for these two known genes could still develop breast cancer due to other genes or risk factors. There are also ethical, legal, social, and insurance issues related to genetic testing that need to be seriously considered before routinely offering and undergoing such testing. Women with positive results might not be able to get insurance, or coverage might be available only at a much higher cost. We strongly recommend that anyone considering undergoing genetic testing talk to a genetic counselor, nurse, or doctor qualified to evaluate your true breast cancer risk and to interpret and explain these test results. It is important to understand and carefully weigh the benefits and risks of genetic testing before these tests are done.

More Common Genes That Might Affect Breast Cancer Risk

There are several common genes, called polymorphic genes, that control the production, metabolism, and utilization of estrogens. We all have these genes—we just inherit different versions of them. Some of the polymorphic gene types occur in small percentages of the population, while others are very common. Some occur more often than others in certain racial or ethnic groups. This may represent older patterns of intermarriage and the resulting gene pool, or it may somehow be closely linked with genes that determine race. Several have been linked to slightly increased risk for breast cancer. Others have been linked to a predisposition to producing high levels of estrogens but may not be related per se to breast cancer risk. These genes may regulate how the body interacts with the environment in determining how hormones will affect the development and growth of breast tumors. Thus, study of these genes is a very important focus of breast cancer research today.

Pregnancy, Menstrual History, and Hormones

If you began menstruating at an early age (before age twelve), you have about a 30 to 40 percent increased risk of developing breast cancer compared with women who got their first menstrual periods after age sixteen. If you have never had a pregnancy lasting six months or more, or you had your first child after age thirty, you are at 50 to 100 percent higher risk for breast cancer compared with women who had their first full pregnancy before age twenty. Breast-feeding, on the other hand, seems to reduce your risk for breast cancer. Women who have breast-fed for the longest total amount of time seem to have the greatest protection. In several studies, women who breast-fed for six months or more reduced their risk for breast cancer by 30 to 40 percent compared with women who had never breast-fed. If you stop menstruating at age forty-five or younger, your risk of getting breast cancer is about half that of a woman who continues menstruating after age fifty-five. This younger age at menopause is protective whether it comes about naturally or through surgical removal of the ovaries. (Hysterectomy or removal of the uterus without removal of the ovaries reduces breast cancer risk only very slightly. The important protective factor of early menopause seems to be the slowdown or removal of ovarian function.)

Blood Hormones

Women whose bodies continue to produce large amounts of estrogen (female hormones) and androgens (male hormones) after menopause have a much higher risk of breast cancer compared with women who produce low levels of these hormones. Although women's ovaries slow down their hormone production after menopause, they continue to produce androgens, which then get converted into estrogens in other parts of the body, especially in fat tissue. Testosterone is an example of such an androgen. Since women who have passed menopause usually have a large amount of fat stores compared to muscle bulk, most of their blood estrogens come from what their body fat produces.

Several studies have measured blood levels of estrogen, androgens, and other hormones in women who eventually developed breast cancer compared with women who did not develop breast cancer. Most of the studies found that women who had high levels of any of the following hormones had an increased risk for developing breast cancer: estrogen, testosterone, other androgens, prolactin, insulin, and insulinlike growth factor. This last hormone is a protein that influences cells in the body to grow, including cancer cells.

Women whose bones are very dense or strong have a higher risk for breast cancer than women with less dense bones. Scientists believe that having highly dense bones is a marker for a lifetime exposure to high levels of estrogen. The estrogen keeps the bones stronger but unfortunately also has potentially harmful effects on the breast. This is not to say that having weak bones is a good thing! (Women with weak bones, or osteoporosis, have a high risk of sustaining fractures, including hip fractures.) Rather, high bone density may be a marker of increased breast cancer risk. If your doctor gives you a test to measure your bone strength (called a DEXA scan) and determines that you have very dense bones, you may also have high levels of blood estrogen. In this case, you might want to avoid hormone replacement therapy so that you do not add estrogen to your body.

Hormone Pills, Shots, and Creams

Taking postmenopausal estrogen replacement increases your risk for breast cancer by about 30 percent. Risk is highest if you have used estrogen therapy for more than five years. If you stop taking estrogen, your risk returns to that of the general population within five years of stopping. Estrogen therapy also increases the dense patterns seen on some women's mammograms—these patterns are associated with increased breast cancer risk. These increased density patterns also make it more difficult for a radiologist to find small cancers, making the mammogram less sensitive at detecting cancer at an early stage in some women. If you have a high risk of developing breast cancer, or if you have had breast cancer, most doctors would advise you to avoid postmenopausal estrogen. Some researchers believe that adding the hormone progesterone to estrogen further increases your risk for breast cancer.

Many women are taking "natural" hormones, or herbs or soy derivatives that have hormonelike properties. Even though you may think that "natural" means safe, you should be aware that we do not know what are the long-term effects of these substances. Some of them may compete with estrogens and may therefore reduce estrogen exposure of breast cells and protect against breast cancer. Others may act just like estrogens and could therefore increase risk for breast cancer. Since so little is known about these compounds, if you are seriously concerned about your risk for breast cancer or are at high risk for breast cancer, you should limit your intake of them and take them for no longer than five years. Small amounts of soy, such as including tofu in a varied diet, should not pose a problem. There are several studies just starting that will provide some information in the next five years or so regarding the breast safety of some of these substances.

Studies on breast cancer and oral contraceptives are still ongoing, but new evidence suggests that any risk from taking the pill is slight, if present at all. Any increase in risk that might be caused by oral contraceptives appears to be limited to women who have used oral contraceptives for many years, who began using them at an early age (i.e., in their teens), or who have a strong family history of breast cancer.

Breast Density

The doctor who reads a mammogram can not only see whether there is a cancer present but can also look at the pattern of structures present in the breast. Breast glands and ducts look like dense patterns on mammograms. In contrast, fat looks clear. Researchers have found that women who have very dense mammogram patterns have a fourfold higher risk for breast cancer compared with women who do not have dense breasts. As women age, their levels of density tend to decrease. Estrogen replacement therapy after menopause tends to increase densities in some women. There are several studies going on to see if there are things that can change women's mammogram patterns. Preliminary evidence suggests that estrogen increases density, while a low-fat diet, Tamoxifen therapy, and exercise decreases density.

Previous Benign Breast Disease and In Situ (Preinvasive) Breast Cancer

If you have had breast lumps in the past, your risk for breast cancer in the future may be higher than if you had not had lumps. "Benign breast disease" is the term for breast lumps that are not cancerous. Some types of benign breast disease increase risk, while most do not. Most fibrocystic changes, fibroadenomas, and cysts do not increase a woman's chances of developing breast cancer. If you had a biopsied lump, and it was a form called proliferative, or if it contained "atypical" cells or "hyperplasia," then your risk for future breast cancer is about two to four times that of women who have never had benign breast disease.

Some breast cancers are detected early, when they are still completely confined to the tiny structures of the breast where they first arose. These are called "in situ" (meaning in the original place) breast cancer. If removed promptly, the cancer has no chance to spread and poses no future risk. However, women who have had in situ breast cancer in the past are up to twelve times more likely to get breast cancer in the future.

Environmental Risk Factors

Radiation in high doses is a strong cancer initiator of breast cells. Women who were exposed to high doses of radiation, as occurred in Hiroshima and Nagasaki in Japan in World War II, had very high rates of breast cancer compared with unexposed women. Women who have had chest area radiation as a child or young woman as treatment for another cancer (such as lymphoma) have a significantly increased risk for breast cancer. Women who in past decades had high exposure to medical X-ray procedures such as fluoroscopy also appear to be at high risk. The increased risk seems to occur only in women who were exposed to radiation before age forty.

The very small doses of radiation present in mammograms do not appear to increase breast cancer risk, and for virtually all women any tiny risk from that radiation is far outweighed by the life-saving effect of mammography in detecting early cancers. In addition, most women do not have mammograms before age forty, so that the radiation from mammograms should not pose a problem.

Some suspected breast carcinogens (cancer-causing substances) include chlorinated hydrocarbons such as the pesticide DDT and PCBs. The pesticides may act as powerful estrogens once in the body, stimulating breast cells to proliferate, that is, to replicate themselves. There are several ongoing studies looking more closely into these environmental contaminants. So far, however, none have been shown to increase the risk for breast cancer. More definitive research results should be available in a few years.

Some studies have indicated that women exposed to large amounts of electromagnetic fields have an increased risk for breast cancer. This increased risk has been observed only in electrical workers. There is no good evidence from scientific studies that exposure typically encountered in the home from appliances increases the risk of breast cancer. If electromagnetic fields do increase risk, it may occur through effects on the pineal gland in the brain, which controls the production and release of melatonin, a hormone that can affect estrogen levels.

Nutrition

High-fat, low-fiber diets, with few fruits and vegetables, have been implicated in increased breast cancer risk, but little has been conclusively proved. Much of our information about diet and breast cancer comes from comparisons across countries. These studies show that women who live in countries with low-fat, high-fruit/vegetable, and high-fiber diets have much lower risk of developing breast cancer, compared with women who live in countries with high-fat, low-fruit/vegetable, and low-fiber diets. Women from the low-risk countries such as Japan and China who immigrate to high-risk countries like the United States tend to take on the high-risk profile of women in their adopted countries. Other clues to a relationship between diet and breast cancer have come from animal studies. Laboratory animals fed diets high in fats of any kind tend to develop more breast cancers than animals fed low-fat diets.

Studies of women in the United States have been less informative, probably because very few American women have diets with a low enough percent of calories from fat to make a difference in their risk. Many nutrition-cancer experts believe that dietary fat must be kept at less than 20 percent of daily calories in order to reduce risk of breast cancer. Another problem with studying women's diets directly is that women who have lower-fat diets tend to also have higher intakes of fruits, vegetables, and fiber. So it is unclear which dietary factors are the most important in controlling risk. It may be that the whole package of a diet that is low-fat, high-fruit/vegetable, and high-fiber will be important for women to adopt.

Alcohol

If you drink two or more alcoholic drinks per day you may have a doubled risk of getting breast cancer, compared with nondrinkers. It doesn't appear to matter what kind of alcohol you drink—all alcohol appears to be associated with increased risk for breast cancer. Alcohol increases the levels of estrogen in the blood, possibly through the toxic effects of alcohol on the liver. Since we know that some aspects of estrogen exposure are related to increased risk for breast cancer, it makes sense that drinking alcohol would increase risk. Alcohol can also depress immune function, which may be important in breast cancer development. A recent analysis from the Nurses' Health Study, a follow-up study of more than 120,000 United States nurses, indicates that folic acid supplementation may help to alleviate the increased risk from alcohol.

Tobacco

Although other types of cancer are more strongly related to tobacco use, recent studies suggest that smoking can also increase the risk of developing breast cancer in some women. The increased risk associated with smoking may be genetically determined.

Body Size and Shape

Researchers have known for many years that women with bigger body size are at higher risk for getting breast cancer than women with smaller body size. Taller women have higher risk than shorter women. On average, women who are 5'8" or taller have one and a half to two times greater risk compared with women who are 5'2" or shorter. Tall women may have higher levels of growth hormones, which might stimulate and promote cancer cell growth. Alternatively, tallness may just be a marker of good nutrition during childhood—perhaps girls with access to large quantities of high-calorie and high-fat foods both grow taller and have higher risk of breast cancer from the types and amounts of foods they ate as children and teens.

Researchers have also long noted an association between increasing weight and breast cancer risk. Most researchers now look at weight corrected for height. The most common measure is called the body mass index, or BMI. The higher your BMI, the higher your risk of getting breast cancer after menopause, the time when most breast cancers occur. Paradoxically, a higher BMI offers some protection against developing breast cancer before you reach menopause. We think that these different associations between BMI and breast cancer risk in younger versus older women are related to hormones. Women who are overweight in their twenties, thirties, and forties are more likely to have irregular menstrual periods and to be ovulating only occasionally, which reflects lower estrogen levels compared with other women of similar ages. On the other hand, women with large amounts of fat stores make estrogen in their body fat, which makes their estrogen levels higher than those of women who are thin. After menopause, this amount of estrogen made in fatter women's body fat is enough to push overweight and obese women into a higher-risk category. The placement of body fat could also be important, as we describe here.

The Nurses' Health Study reported on more than 95,000 nurses who had been asked about their weight and lifetime weight patterns, and were followed for sixteen years for risk for breast cancer. In that study, women who had a BMI of 31 or greater (who were obese) had a 60 percent higher risk for breast cancer than women with a BMI of 20 or less. Women who had gained fifty pounds or more after age eighteen had double the risk for breast cancer compared with women whose weight stayed the same after age eighteen. They also found an interaction between weight and use of hormones, and they estimated that overweight and hormone use accounted for one-third of all of the breast cancer that developed in that study.

The pattern of body fat accumulation may be important in determining risk for breast cancer. Most of the epidemiological studies measured only women's heights and weights, or asked women about their current and past weight. The Iowa Women's Health study, how-

Figure 2.3. Most cancers are caused by a combination of environment and lifestyle.

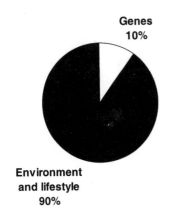

**Genes
10%**

**Environment
and lifestyle
90%**

Graph design by Clayton Hibbert.

ever, obtained measurements of women's waist and hip circumferences. The study asked more than 41,000 women living in Iowa questions about their health and lifestyle habits, and followed them over time to look for occurrences of cancer. The researchers discovered that women who had large waist circumferences had the highest risk for breast cancer, although this was confined to women who had a family history of breast cancer.

Exercise

Recent research suggests a link between regular exercise and reduced risk of developing cancer. We think that the protection that might occur does so through beneficial effects on a woman's hormone production and metabolism. Since this is the major topic of this book, this information is given in great detail in Chapters 5 and 6 and throughout the book.

A Unifying Picture of Breast Cancer Risk

There is convincing evidence that cancer development in breast cells is a two-step process. Something injures the breast cell's DNA, its central structure, such as exposure to radiation or a DNA defect that is inherited in a woman's family, or some other carcinogen. Then some factor, or group of factors, affects the damaged cell to promote the development of cancer. The most likely factors appear to be hormones, either those that a woman's own body makes or those she gets from the environment or from a medication. These hormonal promoters can also be increased by a sedentary lifestyle, a high-fat diet, or even moderate alcohol use. Other factors such as immune status and how well the breast cells can regulate their own growth may also be important in promoting cancer.

Chapters 5 and 6 give you information about a way possibly to reduce your risk of breast cancer through adding regular exercise to your life. Chapter 7 gives you advice on nutrition choices that might protect against breast cancer. Chapter 4 gives you tips on various other things you can do to reduce your risk.

Summary

There are several factors that increase your risk for breast cancer by three to four or more times.

- Being over age sixty-five
- Living in North America or Europe
- Strong family history of breast cancer in three or more close relatives (mother, sisters)
- Having a genetic mutation in a "breast cancer" gene such as BRCA1 or BRCA2
- History of early cancer (such as carcinoma in situ)
- History of certain benign breast diseases (such as proliferative disease with atypia)
- High amounts of density patterns on mammograms
- Exposure to high levels of radiation, such as radioactive fallout

There are several factors that approximately double your risk for breast cancer.

- High blood levels of estrogens and male hormones
- Excessive alcohol intake (more than two alcohol drinks per day)
- Starting menopause at age fifty-five or later
- No pregnancies (of six months' duration or more)
- Late age at first pregnancy (of six months' duration or more)
- History of endometrial or ovarian cancer

Some factors increase your risk by 30 to 70 percent.

- Long-term use of postmenopausal hormone replacement therapy
- Early age at onset of periods
- Never breast-feeding
- Overweight (increases risk after menopause)

- Excessive lifetime weight gain
- Body fat mostly around your waist, rather than your hips and thighs
- Tall height
- Sedentary lifestyle
- Dietary pattern low in fruits, vegetables, or fiber, or high in fat

3

Overview of Breast Cancer
and Its Treatment

You may know people who have had breast cancer. You may have had
breast cancer yourself. No matter what your connection has been with
the disease, there are always new things to learn about breast cancer and
its treatment. More news is good news with this serious disease, as more
advances in treatments are being researched each year. In this chapter,
we give you an outline of breast cancer and its treatment. We describe
breast anatomy. We discuss the various types and stages of breast cancer.
We present some of the testing that is done on breast tumors to help
determine prognosis and optimal therapy. We describe the various treatments for breast cancer in common practice. Finally, we present some of
the new, promising research on breast cancer treatment being conducted at our institutions and around the world.

Breast Anatomy and Breast Cancer

The main components of a female breast are the lobules, or sacs, that
produce milk; the ducts that connect the lobules to the nipple; and the
surrounding fatty tissue. Breast cancer arises in cells lining the insides of
the lobules and the ducts. The fatty tissue of the breast contains ligaments, blood vessels, and lymphatic vessels. Lymphatic vessels carry
lymph, a clear fluid that contains tissue waste products and immune system cells. Cancer cells from the breast may enter lymph vessels and

spread to the underarm lymph nodes, which are small bean-shaped collections of immune system cells. If breast cancer cells reach the lymph nodes under the arm, they are more likely to have spread to other organs of the body as well.

Types of Breast Cancer

Carcinoma in Situ of the Breast

In situ breast cancer is a tumor that is confined to the ducts or lobules of the breast and has not invaded surrounding fatty tissues or spread to other organs of the body. There are two types of in situ breast tumors: lobular carcinoma in situ and ductal carcinoma in situ.

Lobular carcinoma in situ, commonly called LCIS, begins in the lobules but does not penetrate through the lobule walls. Most breast specialists do not consider lobular carcinoma in situ to be a true breast cancer, but women with this diagnosis have a higher risk of later developing a more serious form of breast cancer in either breast.

Ductal carcinoma in situ, commonly called DCIS, is the more common type of in situ breast cancer. Ductal in situ cancer cells inside do

Figure 3.1. Lymph system of the breast

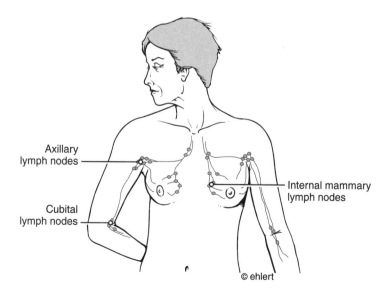

not spread through the walls of the duct into the fatty tissues of the breast or elsewhere in the body. Ductal carcinoma in situ is most commonly diagnosed by finding abnormal calcium deposits, called calcifications, on a mammogram. The calcifications themselves do not represent cancer but signify increased breast cell activity.

Invasive Breast Cancer

Invasive Ductal Breast Cancer

Invasive ductal cancer is the most common form of breast cancer; it accounts for about 80 percent of all breast cancer cases. Some doctors call this type of cancer "infiltrating ductal cancer." This cancer breaks through the wall of the duct to invade into the breast fatty tissue. It can spread to other parts of the body through the lymphatic system and the bloodstream.

Invasive Lobular Breast Cancer

Invasive, or "infiltrating," lobular cancer starts in the lobules of the breast. Like invasive ductal breast cancer, it can spread beyond the breast to other parts of the body. Invasive lobular carcinoma tends to grow in a diffuse, spreading pattern within the fatty tissue of the breast instead of the solid ball pattern that is typical of invasive ductal carcinoma. Therefore, it is frequently more difficult to detect invasive lobular carcinoma with mammography or physical examination at an early stage. Invasive lobular carcinoma is also more likely to occur in both breasts.

Inflammatory Breast Cancer

Inflammatory breast cancer is an uncommon, rapidly growing, aggressive cancer. The skin of the affected breast is red, warm, and thickened with the consistency of an orange peel. These skin changes are due to the spread of cancer cells within the lymphatic channels of the skin.

Stages of Breast Cancer and Treatment Decisions

The stage of breast cancer indicates how far it has spread within the breast, to nearby lymph nodes and other tissues, and to distant organs such as the liver, lungs, and bones. The stage of breast cancer is one of the most important factors doctors use in making treatment recommendations and in predicting prognosis.

Carcinoma in Situ

Treatment of ductal carcinoma in situ usually includes surgery to the breast with or without radiation therapy. Chemotherapy or hormonal treatments are not generally required, and lymph node surgery is not usually performed. The prognosis from ductal carcinoma in situ is excellent: Almost 100 percent of women with this diagnosis are still alive five to ten years after their diagnosis. The main risk of recurrence is in the breast or chest tissue. Clinical studies have shown that tamoxifen may reduce risk of developing a new or recurring breast cancer.

Early Stage Invasive Breast Cancer: Stages I and II

Stage I and II invasive breast cancers are generally considered "early stage." In stage I breast cancer, the tumors is smaller than 1 inch (2 centimeters) in size and the cancer has not spread to the lymph nodes under the arm or other sites beyond the breast. In stage II breast cancer, the tumor is 1 to 2 inches (2 to 5 centimeters) in size or it has spread to the lymph nodes under the arm.

Patients with early stage invasive breast cancer are usually treated initially with mastectomy or lumpectomy. In a lumpectomy, the surgeon removes the cancer and some surrounding tissue but leaves the rest of the breast intact. In a mastectomy, the surgeon removes the entire breast. The surgeon also removes underarm lymph nodes to determine if the breast cancer has spread. Most doctors recommend radiation therapy after breast lumpectomy. Patients may also be treated with chemotherapy or hormone therapies.

Advanced Stage Invasive Breast Cancer: Stage III

Stage III breast cancer is a more advanced cancer, but it has not spread outside of the breast or surrounding tissues or lymph nodes. Patients with advanced stage breast cancer usually are treated with chemotherapy followed by surgery and radiation therapy.

Metastatic Breast Cancer: Stage IV

In stage IV breast cancer, the tumor has spread to distant sites such as the liver, lungs, bones, brain, or lymph nodes outside of the underarm. This type of breast cancer is generally viewed as an incurable disease, although there is wide variation in the number of years that patients may live with this disease. Physicians and researchers are optimistic that some women with stage IV breast cancer may be cured with new forms of treatment.

ℒ☙   Treatments

Several types of special pathology tests can be done on breast cancer tissue removed during surgery or biopsy. These tests can help determine whether the tumor is likely to grow slowly or quickly, whether it is likely to recur, and whether is it likely to respond to certain types of treatment. Some common tests are estrogen and progesterone hormone receptors, HER-2, and cell proliferation.

Breast Surgery

Nearly all women with breast cancer will have some type of surgery. A lumpectomy is an operation to remove only the cancer and the surrounding normal tissue. The goal with a lumpectomy is to remove the cancer without leaving residual cancer cells in the breast. Lumpectomy usually is followed by radiation therapy to destroy any cancer cells that may remain in the breast. Lumpectomy is an option for many women with breast cancer. An operation to remove the breast is a mastectomy. In a simple mastectomy, the entire breast is removed. In a modified radical mastectomy, some axillary lymph nodes are removed along with the breast tissue.

Studies have shown that patients treated with lumpectomy plus radiation have comparable survival to women treated with mastectomy. The decision between a mastectomy and lumpectomy depends on many factors, including the patient's preference, size of the tumor, likelihood that all of the tumor can be removed without removing the entire breast, size of the breast, anticipated cosmetic result, ability to adequately monitor the patient for recurrence after surgery, patient's age and health, and how far a patient lives from a radiation therapy facility.

Lymph Node Surgery

Whether a woman has a mastectomy or lumpectomy, it is important to know whether the cancer involves the lymph nodes under the arm, an indicator of possible spread throughout the body. In most cases of invasive breast cancer, the surgeon also removes lymph nodes under the arm to help determine the stage of disease and plan further treatment. Although the lymph node status provides important information that helps in making recommendations about the need for radiation and chemotherapy, the long-term side effects—lymphedema, nerve injury, and limitations on range of motion—can be uncomfortable and occasionally debilitating. Surgeons are currently investigating a way to reduce the number of axillary lymph node dissections performed in breast cancer patients by using a technique called sentinel lymph node mapping.

Reconstructive Surgery

Breast reconstruction can be done at the same time as the mastectomy or months to years later. Breast reconstruction typically involves either the insertion of a saline implant or a tissue transplant. Saline implants are not thought to impose any risk to the local tissue or to other parts of the body. Tissue transplants involve taking muscle, fat, and skin from the lower stomach, back, or buttock and moving it to the chest area, where it is shaped into the form of a breast. Many women report physical and emotional satisfaction from these types of breast reconstruction, but many women opt not to have this additional surgery.

Radiation Therapy

Radiation can destroy cancer cells left behind in the breast, chest wall, or armpit after surgery. Occasionally it can be used to shrink a tumor before surgery. In most cases, a lumpectomy is followed by radiation therapy, to reduce the risk of local recurrence of the breast cancer within the remaining breast. In some cases, radiation is also recommended following a mastectomy, if there is a high risk of tumor cells remaining behind after surgery. When radiation therapy follows breast surgery, a machine delivers radiation to the breast and chest wall and in some cases to the lymph nodes.

Possible side effects of radiation to the breast or chest wall include fatigue and skin irritation, such as itchiness, redness, soreness, peeling, or darkening of the breast. Changes to the breast tissue and skin usually go away in six to twelve months. In some women, the breast becomes smaller and firmer after radiation therapy. Radiation therapy of underarm lymph nodes can also cause lymphedema. Radiation to the breast does not cause hair loss, vomiting, or diarrhea, nor does it make the patient radioactive.

Chemotherapy and Hormonal Therapy

Therapies that circulate through the body's bloodstream to attack cancer cells wherever they may have spread are called "systemic" treatments. The most commonly used breast cancer systemic therapies are chemotherapy and hormonal therapy.

Systemic treatment given to patients after surgery is called adjuvant therapy. This is aimed at reducing the likelihood of tumor spread and recurrence in the future and increasing the possibility of cure. Adjuvant therapy does not guarantee that distant spread of cancer will not occur in the future, but it does lower the likelihood.

The decision about whether to include adjuvant chemotherapy or hormone therapy in the breast cancer treatment plan weighs the possible benefits to be gained from the treatment with the risks and side effects of the treatment. Many factors are taken into consideration, including the patient's overall health, the stage of the tumor, and the hormone receptor status of the tumor. The pathologic grade of the tumor, DNA studies, and HER-2 studies may also influence the decision about whether a patient may benefit from systemic therapy.

Therapy given before breast surgery is called "neoadjuvant" therapy. This approach is commonly used in larger, more advanced stage breast cancers. If a patient's cancer has already shown signs of spread to distant sites, then systemic neoadjuvant therapy is generally used as the main treatment.

Chemotherapy

Chemotherapy may be given by mouth or by injection into a vein or muscle. The drugs then enter the bloodstream and travel through the body to kill cancer cells that have spread from the original site. Adjuvant chemotherapy has been proved through large clinical trials to improve the cure rate and overall survival for breast cancer patients. Adjuvant chemotherapy may reduce the risk of recurrence in breast cancer by as much as 40 percent.

Chemotherapy is given in cycles—a treatment period followed by a recovery period, then another treatment. Most adjuvant breast cancer chemotherapy regimens include four to six cycles of treatment (usually lasting three to four weeks per cycle). In most cases, breast cancer is treated with a combination of drugs. Common adjuvant breast cancer drugs include doxorubicin (Adriamycin), methotrexate, 5-fluorouracil (5-FU), and cyclophosphamide (Cytoxan), paclitaxel (Taxol), and docetaxel (Taxotere). Most patients undergoing chemotherapy for breast cancer are treated on an outpatient basis in a hospital or clinic.

All adjuvant chemotherapy regimens for breast cancer cause side effects, but most patients are able to do their usual activities most of the time (perhaps at a slower pace). Fatigue is the most common side effect and often is worse near the end of treatment. Many women treated for breast cancer experience little or no nausea, and others benefit from new, improved antinausea medications. The chemotherapy drugs can affect all the blood cells that are made in the bone marrow (white blood cells that fight infection, red blood cells that carry oxygen, and platelets that help stop bleeding). Levels of these blood cells are checked frequently while patients are receiving chemotherapy, and low levels of certain cells may lead to changes in chemotherapy doses, addition of blood cell growth factors, and sometimes blood transfusions. Hair loss, skin and nail changes, changes in bowels, interruption of menstrual cycles, infections, and mouth sores are all potential side effects. Whether a certain symptom will occur depends on the regimen and on the patient. Most of the side effects from chemotherapy are short-term and end after com-

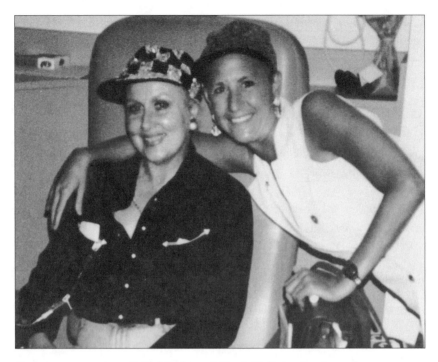

Breast cancer patients Julie Macke and Carol Melis in the chemotherapy infusion room at the University of Washington Cancer Center. Lipstick and a fancy sequined hat helped Julie and Carol look good and feel better while on chemotherapy.

pletion of the chemotherapy treatment. Permanent side effects can include early menopause, rare cases of heart failure from the Adriamycin, and the even rarer development of preleukemia and leukemia years after treatment.

Hormonal Therapy

Estrogen and other hormones can affect the growth of breast cancer cells, like normal breast cells. Hormone therapy for breast cancer may include the use of drugs to change the way that hormones or their receptors work. In premenopausal women, treatment may include surgery or drugs to decrease hormone production by the ovaries. In general, hormone therapy is effective only if the breast cancer cells test positive for either estrogen or progesterone receptor. Like chemotherapy, hormone therapy is a systemic treatment; it attacks cancer cells throughout the body.

The most common hormonal agents used for breast cancer treatment are the antiestrogens such as tamoxifen. Tamoxifen is proved to be an effective adjuvant treatment for breast cancer and can reduce the risk of recurrence by up to 40 percent. It is also effective in the treatment of metastatic cancer. Tamoxifen is a pill that is taken daily by mouth, usually for five years. Tamoxifen can also help prevent osteoporosis and may decrease the risk of heart attack. Evidence suggests that tamoxifen can reduce the chance of developing a second breast cancer by up to 40 percent in breast cancer survivors. Side effects of tamoxifen include hot flashes, psychological effects such as mood swings, and cataracts. Studies show that there is a slight increased risk of endometrial cancer and blood clots for patients on this drug.

There are other types of hormonal therapy for breast cancer. Drugs called third-generation aromatase inhibitors, letrozole (Femara) and anastrozole (Arimidex), are approved for use in metastatic breast cancer and are being investigated in earlier stage cancers. The progestins, including medroxyprogesterone (Megace), are another important class of anti–breast cancer hormonal drugs in advanced breast cancer.

High-Dose Therapy and Stem Cell Transplants

Research has shown that some tumors may respond better to increased levels of chemotherapy, a so-called dose-response level. The effects of these drugs on the bone marrow often limit the dose of chemotherapy that can be given to a patient. High-dose chemotherapy regimens use drug doses five to ten times that given in standard regimens with the hope of overcoming tumor drug resistance and achieving cure. The bone marrow, which is killed or "ablated" by most high-dose chemotherapy regimens, is "rescued" by giving back blood stem cells previously collected from the patient. These stem cells migrate and settle into the patient's bone marrow, where they regenerate the blood cells, including white cells to fight infection, red cells to carry oxygen, and platelets to help with blood clotting.

Results of recent large, randomized clinical trials have shown mixed results with these treatments. The majority of studies reported have shown no improvement in survival for breast cancer patients who underwent transplantation procedures. Since these studies have not yet proved the benefit of transplantation in breast cancer, patients considering undergoing high-dose chemotherapy and stem cell transplantation should do so in the setting of a clinical trial in an experienced medical institution.

✎ New Treatment Strategies in Breast Cancer

Many promising new breast cancer treatments are being developed and investigated in clinical trials. The University of Washington and the Fred Hutchinson Cancer Research Center are pioneering research in the areas of cancer vaccines, gene therapy, apoptosis, and many other exciting biologically oriented treatment approaches.

Drugs That Promote Immune System Attacks on Cancer Cells

This therapy utilizes components of the immune system, our body's defense against infection and cancer, in the treatment program. Antibodies are an important part of our natural immunity. Biologically engineered antibodies directed against certain tumor proteins can be given intravenously, sometimes in combination with drugs or radiation, to target and treat cancer. One of these targets is the HER-2 protein. Trastuzumab (Herceptin), a monoclonal antibody that targets the HER-2 receptor, was approved in 1998 for the treatment of metastatic breast cancer. Herceptin has remarkably little toxicity to normal cells, with proven survival benefit for metastatic breast cancer patients whose tumors have excess amounts of the HER-2 protein. Herceptin is currently being evaluated in earlier stage breast cancer, as well as in other types of tumors.

Another form of immunotherapy under active investigation is vaccine therapy. Tumor vaccination techniques usually target tumor antigens found on the cancer cell surface. Breast cancer clinical trials are investigating HER-2 and other molecules as potential targets for immunization. Tumor vaccine strategies aim to force the body to recognize the tumor cell as "foreign," turning on the immune defense system to aid in fighting the cancer and preventing recurrence.

Drugs to Prevent Cancer Spread to Bones

Bisphosphonates prevent the breakdown of bone and may also prevent bone metastases in breast cancer patients. Alendronate (Fosamax) is a drug in this class commonly used to treat osteoporosis. A similar drug, pamidronate (Aredia), is a more potent intravenous medication that has demonstrated efficacy in preventing complications and decreasing pain in breast cancer patients with bone metastases. Clodronate, a medication that is less potent than pamidronate, is available in Canada and Europe. Bisphosphonates don't directly target tumor cells, but they can delay or potentially prevent spread of tumor in the bones. Large-scale studies are underway to evaluate whether early use of drugs of this type can actually prevent bone metastases from occurring in the first place.

Drugs That Prevent Blood Vessels from Nourishing Tumors

Researchers are trying to understand how cancer cells spread to healthy tissues. A cancer cell must recruit new blood vessels into the area of metastasis in order to continue to receive enough nutrients as the tumor enlarges. Cancer cells secrete substances that stimulate the development of new blood vessels, a process called angiogenesis. Scientists are studying ways of halting this blood vessel development with drugs called angiogenesis inhibitors in the hope that it will prevent cancers from growing and spreading.

Drugs That Promote Cancer Cell Death

Apoptosis is a process by which tumor cells die following exposure to chemotherapy and radiation therapy. All cells in our body are capable of undergoing apoptosis under normal conditions, and our body uses this process in the everyday upkeep and turnover of normal cells. Scientists are working to understand the substances that can stimulate and inhibit this complicated process of cell death. With a better understanding of apoptosis, it may someday be possible to turn on cell death signals specifically in tumor cells.

Drug-Resistance Genes

Breast cancer is often very treatable, but once it has begun to spread, it frequently becomes resistant to chemotherapy and hormone therapy drugs. A previously effective treatment can become ineffective, and some of the tumor cells survive by finding a way to overcome the toxicity of the drug. Scientists are just beginning to understand how cancer cells manage to survive the chemotherapy exposure and develop resistance to chemotherapy. One type of drug resistance is called multidrug resistance, in which cancer cells become unresponsive to a variety of chemotherapy drugs. A number of drugs that inhibit multidrug resistance are being studied in clinical trials.

There is hope in the field of breast cancer treatment. Newer therapies offer the promise of specifically attacking tumor cells while having very low toxicity for normal tissues. A better understanding of the mechanisms by which a breast cancer cell develops, grows, and spreads will allow us to target our treatments to eradicating the cancer while protecting the healthy, normal cells in the body.

Summary

- There are several types of breast cancer. The most important factors predicting prognosis are the size of the tumor and whether it has spread beyond the breast.
- Lobular carcinoma in situ and ductal carcinoma in situ are cancers that have not invaded beyond the breast lobule or duct from which they arose. Prognosis is excellent for both of these types of cancer.
- Stage I or II is considered early breast cancer. Surgery for this stage cancer can include either lumpectomy combined with radiation therapy, or mastectomy.
- There are a number of ways breast cancer is treated, depending

on the patient's preferences, the type of cancer, how far it has spread when diagnosed, and other health conditions of the patient.

- Surgery and radiation treat the cancer cells that are in the breast and underarm lymph nodes. Chemotherapy and hormonal therapy kill cancer cells that have spread beyond the breast and underarm lymph nodes.
- New treatment strategies under study include immunotherapy, drugs to combat metastases to the bone, medications to prevent blood vessels from providing nourishment to tumors, therapy to induce tumor cells to die off, and drugs to overcome tumors that are resistant to therapy.

4

Risk-Reduction Measures
for All Women

Ideally, preventing breast cancer in the first place is better than improving early detection and treatment. Current research on how cell changes can lead to cancer and what factors start, promote, and inhibit these changes gives us hope that in the not too distant future we will be able to prevent it from occurring in many women. The development of cancer is a long process; there are many steps at which we could intervene to prevent cancer from developing. Avoiding exposure to carcinogens (cancer-causing agents) prevents the first step that leads toward cancer—called primary prevention. Most breast cancer prevention research is aimed at stopping the process of cancer development after it has begun—secondary prevention. In this chapter we tell you first how you can determine your risk for breast cancer. We talk about the importance of getting screened regularly for early disease. We suggest ways to avoid potential cancer-causing substances. We give information about things you can change in your life to reduce your risk. Finally, for women at high risk for breast cancer, we offer several alternatives for you to consider for reducing your risk.

There are, unfortunately, no guarantees. Although wearing a seat belt reduces your chance of dying in a car accident, it is not a certainty that you will survive every type of accident. So, too, taking the steps we suggest may help to reduce risk for breast cancer, but they cannot guarantee that you will avoid breast cancer. Similarly, if you do get breast cancer, remember that it is not your fault.

As you saw in Chapter 2, there are many risk factors for breast cancer that could be changed and therefore could provide a means to reduce risk. We call these "modifiable" risk factors. That is, there is something about your health or lifestyle habits that you could change to have a beneficial effect. There is nothing you can do about being female, growing older, or your family history. There are, however, many things you *can* do to change your exercise and dietary habits, alcohol use, and use of hormones. Changing some of these factors can change your biology, in particular what is happening in your body at the level of your cells and connections among cells. This biological change can affect your body's likelihood of developing breast cancer.

How to Determine Your Risk for Breast Cancer: What Are Your Odds?

We have worked with many women who are concerned about their risk for breast cancer. Some have close family members who suffered or died from breast cancer. Some have seen friends deal with the crisis of breast cancer diagnosis or treatment. Others have had one or more breast lumps removed and wonder what this means for their risk of getting breast cancer in the future. Many physicians and researchers also are interested in predicting women's risk of getting breast cancer. For this reason, scientists at the National Cancer Institute and at several research institutes around the country have developed statistical models to predict a woman's risk given her age, family history, and medical and reproductive history. The National Cancer Institute developed an interactive computer program that was distributed to physicians around the country. With this computer program, doctors can estimate a woman's likely chance of getting breast cancer in the next five years and in her lifetime. One reason that they distributed this program to physicians was to help the physician decide if the drug tamoxifen would benefit a particular patient. (We talk more about tamoxifen below.) If you are interested in knowing what this risk estimation program says about your risk, talk to your physician. Or you can request the program (free) from the National Cancer Institute by going to their Web site (see Appendix B).

Your likely risk of getting breast cancer and your own concerns about getting breast cancer will affect how much effort you want to put into prevention. For women who have many relatives with breast cancer, especially if the breast cancer developed at a young age, the risk is higher, and their motivation to take prevention steps will likely be higher. For this reason, we have included a section in this chapter for "high-risk" women.

Finding Breast Cancers Early

The breast is not a vital organ to life. For this reason, if breast cancer is confined to the breast and does not spread, it is not a threat to a woman's life. Breast cancer is a serious invasive cancer, however, and if left unchecked can spread to vital body organs and structures such as the brain, lungs, liver, and bones. When breast cancer spreads to these organs, the result can be significant symptoms that interfere with a woman's everyday quality of life. At the extreme, breast cancer can kill by invading these and other vital organs. The best defense against becoming very sick from breast cancer and dying from it, therefore, is to find cancers early before they have a chance to spread elsewhere in the body.

Mammograms

Screening for breast cancer is the process of searching for cancers before they have had a chance to spread and do damage. The currently available screening techniques for breast cancer are mammograms, breast exam by your doctor or health care provider, and breast self-exam. Regular mammogram screening has been proved to save lives. A screening mammogram is a simple, low-cost X-ray procedure that can reveal breast cancer at its earliest stage, up to two years before it is large enough to be felt. Women who undergo regular mammogram screening (every one to two years) have a 30 to 40 percent lower chance of dying from breast cancer compared with women who do not get regular mammograms. Since about 180,000 women are diagnosed with breast cancer each year, mammograms are saving thousands of lives in the United States yearly. Mammograms don't usually find abnormalities in the breast before they become cancerous, however. For that reason, many researchers are looking for earlier detection tools, with the hope that eventually there will be a blood test or other simple tests that can find cancer cells very early, before they truly become cancerous. Until we have such tests, however, the best strategy is for women age forty and over to have yearly mammograms for the rest of their lives.

The American Cancer Society, the American Medical Association, and the National Alliance of Breast Cancer Organizations recommend the following screening guidelines for all women:

- Have your first screening mammogram at age forty.
- After age forty, have a screening mammogram every year.

Regular mammograms are not recommended for average-risk women under the age of forty in part because the disease is so rare at that age, and in part because younger breast tissue is frequently dense and difficult to read, making mammograms harder to interpret. Women who are at higher than average risk for breast cancer should talk to their health care provider about when to begin having mammograms.

Schedule your mammogram when your breasts will be least tender, such as the week after your menstrual period. Wear a two-piece outfit to make undressing more convenient, and do not use deodorant, perfume, powder, or scented soap that day, as these can affect the film (although

Figure 4.1. Mammogram

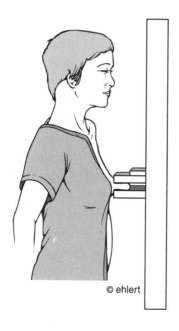

© ehlert

you should follow the instructions of the doctor or clinic that does your mammogram). Bring your prior mammograms (if they were done at another facility) and be prepared with your breast health history. This will help with fast and accurate interpretation of your mammogram results.

Self-Examination

About one in ten breast cancers cannot be spotted on a mammogram. That is why doctors recommend that women also have a yearly breast exam by their physicians or other health care provider. They also recommend that women examine their own breasts each month to look for lumps or thickening. Eighty percent of all breast lumps that are big enough to feel are found by the women themselves. Most of these lumps are not cancer.

When examining your breasts, find a quiet place at home where you will not be distracted. If you are still having your periods, around day 5 of your cycle is the best time to examine your breasts, since breasts are the least lumpy and painful at the conclusion of the menstrual cycle. If you are no longer having periods, pick a day of the month and do your exam on the same day each month. Lie down on your back with a pillow under your back on the side you will be examining. Using the pads of your fingers, not your nails, palpate all of your breast tissue, including your underarm area. Then, stand in front of a mirror and look at your breasts with your arms raised and then with your arms by your sides. You are looking for any changes in your breast or nipple, including new retraction of the nipple, dimpling of the skin, or other skin changes. Some women find that they are better able to palpate their breasts in the shower or bath with soapy hands. The most important thing to remember about breast self-exam is to do it regularly. Don't be afraid of finding something, or having trouble figuring out what is normal. The more you examine your breasts over time, the more familiar you will become with their contours. *Any* change should be followed up with your health care provider.

In addition to getting your yearly mammogram and doing regular breast examinations, there are several things you can do to reduce your risk of getting breast cancer. Most of this book is focused on how you can

Figure 4.2. Breast self-exam

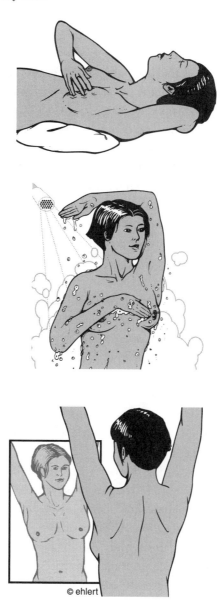

use physical activity and exercise to reduce your risk. This chapter gives you tips on other strategies for risk reduction.

Avoid Cancer-Causing Substances and Agents

When you have X rays taken at your dentist's office, the technician puts a heavy apron on you that covers the front of your body. This is to protect your body's organs that are particularly susceptible to the effects of radiation exposure. Women's breasts are very susceptible to large amounts of radiation. More women who were exposed to the atomic bomb fallout in Hiroshima and Nagasaki, for example, developed breast cancer compared with women who were not exposed. For your own breast health, you should avoid excessive exposure to radiation. If you work in a job where you are exposed to radiation, make sure that you wear your shields and do not exceed the maximal exposure allowed for your job. Do not ask your doctor for X rays that are not necessary to make a diagnosis. For example, if you go to your doctor for a cold, and he or she does not think you need a chest X ray for a diagnosis, do not insist on one. If you live in an area of the country where radon is present in the earth and leaks into basements, have your basement evaluated for radiation. (If there is radon in your house, one solution is to build a finished basement, which contains the radon leakage.) Radon per se has not been linked to breast cancer, but it is known to cause cancers of the lung and other organs.

Decrease Your Intake of Alcohol

You say no to alcohol during the day when you need to be functioning at full steam and don't want your reaction time or thinking ability to be diminished. You avoid alcohol when you will be driving, since you do not want to cause harm to yourself or to others. Protecting your breasts and your general health is another excellent reason to say no to that second glass of wine. Alcohol increases estrogen levels, making more estrogen available to the breast cells and depressing immune function. Alcohol interferes with the absorption of nutrients that can be protective of your breasts and health in general, such as vitamins and minerals. Alcohol damages the liver and could increase the release of liver toxins into the bloodstream. Some of these toxins could be cancer causing. If you can avoid alcohol entirely, that may be the best idea. However, you should at least limit yourself to no more than two alcohol drinks per day.

One study suggests that for women who drink large amounts of alcohol, taking folate supplements might in part counteract the adverse effects of alcohol on the breasts. This is just one study, however. The safer alternative is to avoid excess alcohol. There are other reasons for women to take folate, including reduced risk for birth defects and for protection against heart disease. Moreover, there do not appear to be known adverse effects from folate supplementation.

Limit Your Use of Estrogen and Progesterone Medications

Studies have fairly consistently found that use of estrogen or progesterone hormone replacement therapy for more than five years after menopause increases risk for breast cancer. This leads us to suggest that if you have concerns about your breast cancer risk, you should not use hormone replacement therapy for more than five years. If you use hormones, you should use the lowest possible dose. Depending on what other concerns you have about menopause and the diseases that follow it, you might also consider taking tamoxifen (which has been shown to reduce breast cancer occurrence by up to 50 percent) or raloxifene (which may also reduce breast cancer occurrence).

Hormone therapy after menopause has many benefits, however, so you should talk fully with your physician before you decide for or against hormone therapy. If your main menopausal symptoms are vaginal dryness or related vaginal or urethral conditions, a vaginal estrogen cream may be all that you need. Some amount of estrogen is absorbed into your bloodstream from vaginal estrogen creams, but the level should be lower than from taking an estrogen pill. If your main symptom is an occasional hot flash, you might use mechanical cooling tricks to make you more comfortable. These include wearing wicking clothes such as CoolMax, dressing in layers, and opening windows or doors during a hot flash. This latter will require some understanding on the part of those you live with.

If your main reason for considering hormone therapy is that you are worried about heart disease risk, there are many ways to lower your risk for heart disease other than hormone therapy. Increased aerobic exercise; a low-fat, low-cholesterol, high-fiber diet; weight reduction; low-dose aspirin; stopping smoking; and medications to control high cholesterol and hypertension are all excellent ways to reduce risk of coronary heart disease. Some of these, namely the exercise, diet, and weight control recommendations, are also excellent ways to protect your breasts, giving you added protection from adopting these lifestyle changes.

Think About Planning Your Family Earlier

Several of the reproductive breast cancer risk factors are modifiable in the sense that it is possible to change them. Having your first full-term pregnancy before age twenty-five lowers your risk compared to what it would be if you waited until after you were thirty years old. For many women, however, it is not a simple matter to have their children at a young age. You need to take into account all of the aspects of your life and those around you. Can you afford to start a family now? Do you have the emotional and physical support you need? Do you have some schooling or training to complete before you want to have children? What have you decided as a couple about timing of your children? If, however, all things are equal to you and you are just waiting for the "right time," then for your own health you could consider having your children sooner rather than later. If you have already had your family, you might suggest to your daughters some things to reduce their risk, and having children early can be one recommendation.

When you do have children, breast-feeding them for at least six months will benefit your health and your baby's health. Breast-feeding all of your children for at least six months may reduce your risk for breast cancer by as much as half compared to what your risk would be if you never breast-fed at all. That's as much protection as you'd get from taking tamoxifen, and without any appreciable risks! Breast-feeding provides the best nourishment for your baby, makes feeding at night much easier than getting up to make and heat a bottle, and helps you bond closely with your baby. Breast-feeding is something that almost all women can do, as long as they can bear children. If you can, try to keep breast-feeding each baby for a year or longer. In primitive cultures, babies are breast-fed for two years or longer! In our culture, many moms and babies do not tolerate very long periods of breast-feeding, but the longer you can do it the better.

Adopt a Healthy Lifestyle

Increased exercise, weight control, and improved nutrition are major lifestyle changes you can make that may have powerful effects on reducing your risk. We talk much more about exercise, weight control, and nutrition throughout the rest of the book.

Make Choices About Medications to Prevent Breast Cancer

Scientists around the world are examining the effectiveness of "chemoprevention," using chemicals or drugs to reduce breast cancer risk. Several different medications are under different stages of development and testing. We will talk about only the ones that have undergone, or are undergoing, widespread testing.

In the United States, tamoxifen (trade name Nolvadex), a hormonal therapy that is widely used in the treatment of breast cancer, has been tested as a chemopreventive agent. Researchers have known for some time that women who take tamoxifen for breast cancer have fewer second breast cancers, and they have suspected that women without breast cancer but who are at high risk for developing the disease could also benefit by taking tamoxifen.

In 1998, the National Cancer Institute published results of the National Surgical Breast and Bowel Project's Breast Cancer Prevention Trial, which was a study of more than 13,000 women at risk for developing breast cancer. The study compared breast cancer incidence in high-risk women taking tamoxifen for five years with those taking a placebo (a pill containing no medication). Women were eligible for that study if they were age sixty-two or older, or if they had characteristics that placed them at high risk for breast cancer. This study showed that women at high risk for breast cancer are about 50 percent less likely to develop the disease (at least in the short term) if they take tamoxifen. If you are age sixty-two or older, or otherwise are at high risk for breast cancer, you could benefit from tamoxifen therapy in terms of reduced risk for breast cancer. For women at low or moderate risk for breast cancer, the risks associated with tamoxifen may outweigh its benefits. You will not be able to take both tamoxifen and hormone therapy, so you need to choose one or the other. There are some risks associated with tamoxifen therapy, including some increased risk for endometrial (uterine) cancer, blood clots in the legs or lungs, and stroke. The risks of these conditions are small, however. Endometrial cancer is not a risk if you have had a hysterectomy. If you still have your uterus and decide to take tamoxifen, you should have a yearly test of your uterus lining to be sure that you are not at risk for endometrial cancer. You can lower your risk for blood clots in your legs and lungs by keeping your body weight down and by avoiding long periods of immobility. For example, if you are planning a long car ride, you should stop and get out of the car to stretch and move your legs once every hour or so. Women taking tamoxifen commonly experience hot flashes and vaginal discharge. If you are at high risk for breast cancer, or for developing a second breast cancer, you should discuss chemoprevention strategies such as tamoxifen with your doctor.

Raloxifene (trade name Evista) is similar to tamoxifen except that it

Figure 4.3. Effects of tamoxifen on various diseases (NSABP P-01 Breast Cancer Prevention Trial)

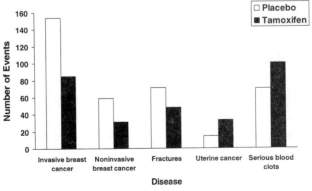

Graph design by Clayton Hibbert.

does not seem to have an adverse effect on the endometrium. It is not clear if it really reduces risk for breast cancer. For that reason, the National Cancer Institute and the National Surgical Breast and Bowel Project are conducting a study to compare raloxifene with tamoxifen, to see if raloxifene has the same protective effect as tamoxifen. If you have passed menopause either naturally or through surgery, and if you are either over age sixty-two or have risk factors for breast cancer (i.e., a family history of breast cancer in close relatives, a certain type of benign breast disease, or a high-risk reproductive history), you may be eligible for this study, which is enrolling patients until 2003–2004. You can learn more about this study, called the STAR trial, by calling their number or visiting their Web site (see Appendix B).

In Italy, fenretinide, a retinoid (a chemical similar to vitamin A), has been tested in 2,972 women age thirty to seventy who have had cancer in one breast to see if their risk of second breast cancers is reduced. The patients were randomly assigned to take either fenretinide or placebo and followed for a median of eight years. Although retinoids can be toxic in high doses, there is evidence that they are effective in preventing skin, oral, bladder, and cervical cancers. Newly published results from the Italian study suggest that fenretinide may lower risk of second cancers in premenopausal women. However, it appeared to have no effect in postmenopausal women.

For High-Risk Women

If you come from a family in which three or more related family members have had breast cancer, you may belong to a high-risk group. Other high-risk women include those known to have a breast cancer gene such as BRCA1 or BRCA2, or who have had a previous breast cancer in one breast, or who have had a biopsy showing lobular carcinoma in situ (LCIS, a precancerous lesion).

Prophylactic Mastectomy

Some women who have several close relatives with breast cancer and face their own probability of getting breast cancer decide to undergo surgical removal of their breasts. In this procedure, known as prophylactic mastectomy, one or both breasts are removed before there is any known breast cancer. When the surgeons remove breasts, they usually follow it with reconstructive surgery so that the woman is left with new breasts made from a combination of artificial materials (like saline implants) and tissue from other parts of her body grafted onto the new breasts.

Drastic as this seems, women who choose this route are for the most part satisfied with their decision. A new publication from the Mayo Clinic reported on 639 women with a family history of breast cancer who underwent this surgery between 1960 and 1993 and were followed for a median of fourteen years. The study showed that women having this surgery cut their risk of dying from breast cancer by almost 90 percent compared to what would have been expected statistically and also compared to what occurred in the women's sisters who did not have a prophylactic mastectomy. This degree of protection is higher than any other method we currently have.

Prophylactic mastectomy is not the only solution for women at high risk for breast cancer. It is true that some women with BRCA gene mutations will develop a very aggressive breast cancer at a young age, and a prophylactic mastectomy might add many years to their life expectancy. However, some women with BRCA gene mutations will never develop breast cancer, so they would not benefit from surgery. Still others might develop breast cancer that is found at an early stage by mammography or breast examination and be treated and cured; these women's life expectancy would not be affected by prophylactic mastectomy either. While the operation reduces the risk of breast cancer, it doesn't guarantee that the cancer won't develop in the small amount of breast tissue remaining after the operation.

If you are in a high-risk group and are considering having your breasts removed surgically, you should talk with a genetic counselor and with a breast surgeon to find out what are your options. Most experts also recommend that you get a second opinion before making the decision to have prophylactic breast surgery. After careful deliberation, this might be the right choice for some women.

Prophylactic Oophorectomy

Women who carry the BRCA1 or BRCA2 gene have an increased risk of developing ovarian cancer compared with other women. For this reason, many experts recommend that these women consider having both ovaries removed after they have completed their families. Removal of both ovaries may also protect against breast cancer. In a recent small study, women with the BRCA1 or BRCA2 gene who opted for surgical removal of their ovaries reduced their risk of developing breast cancer by half. Removal of both ovaries in young women causes a drastic reduction in estrogen levels (postmenopausal women's ovaries have stopped producing estrogen). Removal of the ovaries in young women carries some risk, besides the small risk from the surgery itself. The large drop in estrogen levels can lead to cholesterol abnormalities, heart disease, osteoporosis, fractures, severe hot flashes, night sweats, vaginal dryness, and increased vaginal and bladder infections. Most women having their ovaries removed to reduce breast cancer risk do not take estrogen replacement therapy (the whole reason for the ovary removal is to decrease estrogen!). If you know or suspect that you have the BRCA1 or BRCA2 gene, have a frank discussion with your doctor about the benefits and risks of this type of surgery.

Tamoxifen

As we described above, tamoxifen was found in the American study to cut the risk of breast cancer by over 40 percent in high-risk women. If you have a prophylactic mastectomy or oophorectomy, it is not clear that you would also need to take tamoxifen. Talk with your doctor about the benefits and risks of tamoxifen for you. This is a conversation that you should repeat at intervals with your physician, since your chance of developing breast cancer changes with age, and the risks from tamoxifen therapy also change with age.

Summary

- You can estimate your risk for breast cancer by using the Breast Cancer Risk Assessment Tool from the National Cancer Institute.
- You can lower your chances of dying of breast cancer by getting regular yearly mammograms starting at age forty.
- You can reduce your risk of developing breast cancer by:
  — Avoiding cancer-causing substances such as excess radiation (mammograms are okay)
  — Limiting your intake of alcohol
  — Limiting your use of estrogen and progesterone after menopause
  — Having children early, rather than later
  — Breast-feeding your children for six months or more each
  — Avoiding excess weight gain after age eighteen
  — Doing at least thirty minutes daily of moderate- to high-intensity aerobic exercise (such as brisk walking, jogging, fast bicycling)
  — Following a healthful diet (low fat, high fruits and vegetables, high fiber)
  — Considering taking tamoxifen in place of estrogen therapy after menopause

5

Exercise to Reduce Risk— What the Research Shows

There is increasing scientific evidence that regular physical activity is associated with a reduced risk for breast cancer. Thousands of women with and without breast cancer around the world have been interviewed about their exercise habits, and the consistent conclusion is that exercise is an important weapon that women can use to help lower their chance of getting breast cancer. In this chapter we describe the many scientific studies that have linked increased exercise to a reduced risk for breast cancer. We present the scientific findings concerning the association between increased weight and increased risk for most breast cancer. We describe the relationship of weight distribution in risk for breast cancer. By putting these studies together, we give you the big picture of the associations among exercise, body fat, lifetime weight changes, and risk for breast cancer.

The Obesity Factor

For some time, scientists have known that women who are obese have a 30 to 100 percent increased risk of developing breast cancer, compared with thinner women. This increased risk is seen only for breast cancer that develops after menopause, which is the time when most women develop breast cancer. In several epidemiological studies, gaining weight throughout adulthood appeared to be especially dangerous in terms of breast cancer risk. The Nurses' Health Study is collecting data and following more than 121,000 United States nurses who were age thirty to fifty-five years when they joined the study. The Nurses' Health Study researchers found that women who gained more than twenty pounds since age eighteen had a 50 to 100 percent increased risk for breast cancer compared with women who did not gain weight during adulthood. This increase in risk was seen only in women who were not currently using postmenopausal hormone therapy. The increased risk from hormone therapy appeared to overwhelm any effect of weight.

Doctors say that a woman is overweight if her body mass index (BMI) is higher than 25 and obese if her BMI is higher than 30. We describe how to determine your BMI in Appendix A.

Your Body Shape May Be Key

The body area where a woman's fat is deposited may be critical. In the Iowa Women's Health Study, researchers found that women who have an "apple" shape, those who gain fat predominantly around their waist and abdomen, are at higher risk for breast cancer than women who gain fat mostly in the hip and thigh area. Scientists don't know why this is true, but they do know that the fat deposited in the waist and abdominal areas is more active in metabolism and is highly related to risk of other diseases, such as diabetes and heart disease.

Exercise Reduces Body Fat, Especially Around the Middle

The relationship between obesity and breast cancer has led to the question of whether exercise, which reduces body fat, might protect against the development of breast cancer. Exercise is a particularly effective way to take off fat in the internal waist and abdominal areas, that is, the fat that surrounds the internal organs. These internal fat areas are often harder to reduce using diet alone.

Epidemiological Studies of Breast Cancer and Exercise

More than two dozen epidemiological studies have investigated the association between physical activity and breast cancer. Epidemiological studies involve looking at actual individuals who get a disease and comparing them with individuals who do not get the disease. For example, epidemiological studies gave the first clues to an association between family history of breast cancer and the likelihood of an individual getting breast cancer.

In fifteen epidemiological studies of exercise and breast cancer, scientists asked breast cancer patients about their recent and lifetime exercise habits and compared their answers to those of women without breast cancer. Scientists in other epidemiological studies identified large groups of women who exercise regularly, along with comparison groups of sedentary women, and followed both groups to see which were more likely to get breast cancer. In all but three of the studies, breast cancer patients were noted to have exercised less often and for shorter duration, compared to women without breast cancer. This difference was seen both in exercise activities shortly before breast cancer developed and in exercise activities in youth, such as high school and college athletics.

Physical Activity on the Job

Two studies compared women working in various occupations in the state of Washington and in Shanghai, China. The studies found that women who worked in occupations with high levels of physical activity had lower rates of breast cancer and few deaths from breast cancer compared with women in sedentary occupations.

A study in the state of Washington found that women who worked in occupations that required high levels of physical activity on the job had an approximately 30 percent lower risk of dying from breast cancer compared with women who worked in sedentary occupations. Examples of jobs with higher demands of physical activity are housecleaning, nursing, and gardening. Sedentary jobs include office workers and any job that requires sitting or standing for the majority of the time.

Chinese women in Shanghai who spent less than one day a week sitting at their job had a rate of breast cancer occurrence that was about one-third less than that of women who spent more than four days a week sitting down at their job. Similarly, women whose jobs required them to be more active (frequently walking quickly or doing heavy work requiring two arms) also had a one-third reduction in risk compared with women whose jobs required only light activity (sitting with only hand movement or light arm movement).

One problem with this type of study is that the researchers did not determine the total amount of exercise the women were doing, both at work and at home. They simply assumed that the women working in a certain job did the average amount of physical activity usually done at that job. Also, women in certain occupations may be exposed to other cancer-causing agents, such as chemicals or pesticides. Although these possible biases may have existed in these studies, the fact that the researchers did find an association between sedentary jobs and getting breast cancer indicates that more detailed study is needed.

College Athletes

Three studies, two in the United States and one in Finland, have followed several thousand female college athletes for up to seventy years and have found that the athletes had a lower risk of eventually getting breast cancer than did the nonathletic collegiates. Dr. Rose Frisch pioneered such research efforts in exercise and cancer. She sent questionnaires to more than 5,000 female college alumnae; about half were former athletes. She found that the former athletes had a 33 percent lower risk of getting breast cancer compared with the nonathletic women. Finnish researchers gathered information on 1,499 physical education teachers and 8,619 language teachers from 1920 to 1973. The physical education teachers were assumed by the nature of their jobs to be more physically active than the language teachers were. Among women who had not yet gone through menopause, breast cancer occurred less often in the physical education instructors than in the language teachers. For older women, no reduction in risk was seen.

A study of 1,566 University of Pennsylvania alumnae focused on activity patterns during college and followed the women for up to thirty-one years. The researchers found that women who expended 1,000 calories or more per week in sports in college had about half the risk of developing breast cancer after menopause, compared with women who expended fewer than 500 calories per week. This finding persisted even when the researchers controlled for body weight.

These studies give some evidence that exercise at an early age may be important in the exercise-cancer link. This type of study gives some information about the effect of exercise early in life on later risk of breast cancer development. It does not, however, tell us anything about associations between lifetime and recent physical activity levels and breast cancer occurrence.

Recreational Activities and Housework

Studies in the United States

Several studies of exercise and breast cancer risk have gathered information about the types of exercise done by women during recreational and household activities. At the Fred Hutchinson Cancer Research Center in Seattle, Dr. Anne McTiernan and her colleagues have analyzed information collected from 537 breast cancer patients and 492 women without breast cancer. These women were from fifty to sixty-four years of age, a time when breast cancer is often first diagnosed. The study showed that moderate or strenuous aerobic exercise in recent years was associated with a 30 percent reduction in the risk of developing breast cancer. The effect of exercise was still present after the effects of diet and weight difference between exercisers and nonexercisers were taken into account.

A study by Dr. Leslie Bernstein in southern California looked at the lifetime exercise patterns in young breast cancer patients (age forty and under) and in similar-aged women without breast cancer. Women who spent more than about four hours per week exercising reduced their risk of getting breast cancer by 60 percent. This means that exercisers cut their risk of getting breast cancer by more than half.

Rural women who exercise in the teenage years may also have a reduced risk of breast cancer. In 1995, Dr. Robert Mittendorf and his colleagues published results of a study that included 6,888 breast cancer

Figure 5.1. Exercise lowers risk of breast cancer.

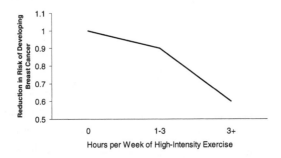

Graph design by Clayton Hibbert.

patients and 9,539 women without breast cancer from Maine, western Massachusetts, New Hampshire, and Wisconsin. All of the women were between the ages of seventeen and seventy-four. The researchers interviewed the women about their participation in strenuous physical activity or team sports from age fourteen to twenty-two. They asked what kind of activities they did, how often they did them, and how long they usually exercised. Women who had exercised vigorously at least once a day in their teenage years had half the risk of getting breast cancer, compared with women who reported doing no strenuous physical activity in their teenage years.

Researchers analyzed data on physical activity and breast cancer from the Nurses' Health Study twice. The first report, published in 1998 by Dr. Rockhill and her colleagues, looked at physical activity patterns in the 85,364 women who had completed relevant forms as of 1980. In that analysis, the researchers looked at the women's reported activity at just one period in time, and they did not find a significant association between level of physical activity and risk of developing breast cancer. In a second analysis of a separate group of nurses published in late 1999, the researchers looked at the women's exercise habits over a span of sixteen years. They found that women who exercised at a moderate or intense level for an hour a day had almost a 20 percent lower risk of getting breast cancer compared with sedentary women. In that study, it did not seem to matter whether the activity was at a moderate or an intense level. They also found that the effect of exercise was the same regardless of body mass index, weight change over time, age, use of oral contraceptives, use of hormone therapy, and family history of breast cancer. Of the women who did exercise, the most common activity was walking; it accounted for 40 percent of all moderate or vigorous exercise hours in this cohort of nurses.

A study was published in 1999 of more than 1,000 breast cancer patients age fifty-five to sixty-four and a similar number of same-age women without breast cancer in Los Angeles, California. The researchers found that women who had exercised at moderate levels for four or more hours per week during their lifetime had approximately half the risk of developing breast cancer compared with sedentary women. Women who exercised at the most vigorous levels had the most protection, and the protection was limited to women who did not gain weight, or gained less than 17 percent of their body weight, during adulthood.

Studies in Other Countries

A large study in Italy confirmed the results of these American studies and found that physical activity in adulthood was more protective against breast cancer than physical activity in adolescence. Dr. Barbara D'Avanzo and her colleagues studied 2,569 Italian breast cancer patients and 2,588 hospital patients without cancer. These researchers discovered that women who exercised more than seven hours per week when they were in their thirties to fifties had a 25 to 35 percent decrease in risk of having breast cancer. Exercise was associated with the same reduction in risk regardless of body size and dietary habits, and whether the women had gone through menopause. The scientists concluded that 36 percent of breast cancer cases in Italy could be prevented if all women increased their physical activity to more than seven hours per week.

Australian women who exercise also appear to have lower risk for breast cancer compared with sedentary women. Australian researchers compared the exercise habits of 451 breast cancer patients of all ages with healthy women. They found a significant decrease in occurrence of breast cancer among women who expended more than 4,000 calories each week in exercise compared with sedentary women. This amount of energy expenditure would be similar to an average-size woman walking about forty-five minutes each day, plus engaging in a vigorous activity such as fast bicycling or aerobics for about three hours per week.

A very large, well-designed study in Norway conducted by Dr. Inger Thune interviewed more than 25,000 women between 1977 and 1983 about their exercise habits at recreation and at work, and followed them over time for an average of thirteen years. They found a significant 37 percent reduction in risk of breast cancer among women who reported exercising regularly at a high level of intensity. The reduction in risk was greatest among lean women, women under the age of forty-five, and women who continued to exercise regularly over a period of three to five years at the beginning of the study. The strengths of this particular study were its large size, its design in following women over time, and taking into account other lifestyle factors such as age, obesity, diet, and pregnancy history.

The Journal of the National Cancer Institute published in 2000 the results of a Netherlands study of more than 900 young women (age twenty-nine to fifty-four) with breast cancer and a similar number of same-age women without breast cancer. The researchers found that women who were more active than their peers when they were age ten to twelve, and who engaged in recreational physical activity, had about one-third lower risk of developing breast cancer compared with women who were sedentary at those ages. Women who started exercising after age twenty had as much protection as women who started in their childhoods or teens. The protection was greatest among women who were lighter; women who were heavy did not appear to have much reduction in risk with recreational physical activity.

Japanese women who are more physically active may also be at reduced risk for breast cancer at any age. In one study, women who exercised for health two or more times per week had a statistically significant 25 percent reduction in risk of developing breast cancer either before or after menopause. This lowering of risk was evident even after the scientists took other risk factors into account, such as age, body fat, and pregnancy history. In another Japanese study, women who engaged in regular sports activity (expending 800 calories or more per week) cut their risk for breast cancer by 70 percent, and women who were very physically active on the job reduced their risk by half compared with sedentary women.

The effect of physical activity on the breast may occur at an early stage in the development of breast cancer. A recent preliminary report of 3,640 Norwegian women between the ages of forty and fifty-six who were receiving regular mammograms indicated that women who exercised more had lower levels of breast tissue density. Lower density level has been found to be associated with a lowered risk of getting breast cancer.

Challenges to Epidemiological Studies of Exercise and Breast Cancer

All of the epidemiological studies have been observational studies. That is, the researchers asked women about their physical activity habits and compared the answers of breast cancer patients with those of women without breast cancer. In a *cohort study*, a large number of healthy persons are asked about their habits at one time and then followed forward in time so that the researchers can study those who eventually develop disease and compare them to those who remain healthy. The Nurses' Health Study, the Iowa Women's Health Study, and the Women's Health Initiative Observational Study are cohort studies. In these studies, women are contacted every year or two and asked to report if they have had any illness or hospitalizations. In some cohort studies the exposures of interest, in this case exercise and physical activity, are asked about every year or two to look at the effects of change on the illness under study. A second type of observational epidemiological study is a *case-control study*, in which individuals with the disease (in this case breast cancer) are asked about exposures and health habits and compared to a sample of individuals without the disease (these latter are called "controls"). There are several ways to collect these samples of breast cancer patients and controls. At the Fred Hutchinson Cancer Research Center, we do many case-control studies in which cancer patients are identified through a population registry, and controls are identified by random phone calls to the general population of the Seattle area. This minimizes the risk of either the cases or controls being a biased sample. Both cohort and case-control studies suffer from some problems of observational studies, but the degree of problem differs between the study type.

One challenge in studying physical activity is that we depend on what a woman tells us about her physical activity habits. She may have trouble recalling what she has done in the past. If we want to know about exercise done in childhood or adolescence, it can be difficult for a woman to recall exactly what she did in those early years. From our own experience, interviews and questionnaires that ask about early life events can be very time-consuming and tiring for the study participants. This fatigue can result in less accurate information. Some women do not feel comfortable "admitting" their sedentary lifestyle and therefore may give misleading answers in order not to feel embarrassed in front of an interviewer. If the questionnaire asks about the intensity of exercise (how hard is the exercise), the answers depend on women's subjective reactions to how "hard" they exercise.

Some researchers neglect to ask about all aspects of a woman's life in which physical activity may be prominent. For example, some women exert a great deal of energy at low- and moderate-level physical activities such as housework and gardening. If the questionnaire or interview does not ask about these activities, then the researcher will underestimate the amount of activity done by these women.

New research indicates that some individuals expend a considerable amount of energy in their minute-to-minute body movements. You've probably noticed that some of your friends seem always to be moving— they shake their legs as they type, move around during meetings, use frequent hand gestures, or seem to have trouble sitting back and relaxing. This type of movement, sometimes called "nervous energy," expends enough energy to keep these individuals thinner than their calmer relatives and friends. It is very difficult to measure this energy expenditure reliably, but by not capturing this type of activity, researchers will underestimate energy expenditure in these individuals.

A difficult piece of the weight–obesity–breast cancer puzzle is that women who are obese are actually protected against breast cancer before menopause. We think that this is because obese women have hormonal abnormalities that prevent or delay ovulation. Their estrogen levels may actually be lower at some times of the month than they would be if they were slimmer. This protection disappears, however, as soon as the obese women reach menopause. As we describe in Chapters 6 and 8, obese women after menopause make estrogen in their fat cells, which increases their risk for breast cancer. Obese women are less likely to exercise at high levels compared with thin women. For these reasons, a study that looks at exercise and risk of breast cancer in young women may not show a protective effect against breast cancer unless the study looks separately at obese and nonobese women.

A serious gap in the knowledge about physical activity and breast cancer is that most of the studies have been conducted with white women. While white women do have the highest overall risk of breast cancer in the United States, women of all races and ethnic backgrounds are at risk for this disease. African-American women have the highest rate of premenopausal breast cancer of any racial or ethnic group in this country and are the most likely to die from the disease if they get it. Many American minority women are overweight or obese and sedentary, and they are getting fatter and more sedentary. If exercise could reduce risk of breast cancer, it could have important public health implications for minority as well as nonminority women. However, without research on women from all racial and ethnic backgrounds, we cannot say for sure what effect exercise will have on risk for all women.

One final question is whether one can do too much exercise, whether extremes of exercise could actually increase rather than decrease risk of breast cancer. You may know women who were competitive athletes when they developed breast cancer, and may well ask, "If she got breast cancer even though she trained heavily every day, how can exercise reduce anyone's risk?" We don't know why some women get breast cancer even though they have no family history of breast cancer and they "do everything right" (keep thin, eat healthy diets, avoid alcohol, exercise, don't smoke, avoid environmental contaminants and pesticides, don't take extra estrogen, had their babies at a young age and breast-fed them, etc.). One theory about trained athletes is that if a woman overtrains, she may actually reduce her immunity, which could increase her risk for cancer at the same time that it increases risk for infections. This is just speculation, however, and should not deter any woman from training and competing in athletics. But all athletes should be aware of the dangers of overtraining and should seek the advice of a sports-medicine physician if they are intent on a longer or more intense training schedule than they are accustomed to.

Putting It All Together

To summarize these important research findings, most of the epidemiological evidence points to an association between decreased risk for breast cancer with increasing levels of physical activity. While a small number of studies did not agree, more than a dozen well-designed and -conducted studies support this association. Epidemiological studies don't always give the same results—some vary just due to chance. Epidemiologists make conclusions about risk factors based on the preponderance of evidence from many studies, just as we have done here. We believe that the evidence is strong but that there are still many questions to be answered about the ability of exercise to prevent breast cancer.

Women who choose on their own to exercise are very different from women who do not choose to exercise. Several studies have shown that women who exercise also have other good health habits. They tend to drink less alcohol, eat healthier diets, smoke less if at all, take more vitamin supplements, and take better overall care of their health. So when we study women who exercise and compare them to women who do not exercise, we can never be completely sure that the exercise by itself is having the effect.

There are several pieces of evidence, however, that point to exercise as an important way to reduce risk for breast cancer. First, exercise delays the onset of menstrual periods. Second, exercise reduces levels of blood estrogens in the adolescent and adult years. Third, exercise maintains a healthy body weight and reduces the amount of fat gain over the lifespan. Fourth, exercise is key to preventing weight gain after diet-induced weight loss. Fifth, exercise promotes a healthy immune system, which may help to fight cancerous cells so they never develop into a full-blown tumor. Chapter 6 covers in detail the biological mechanisms by which exercise may protect the breasts against cancer.

You may have some specific questions about the relationship between exercise and breast cancer. Scientists may not have the answers to many of these questions. Based on what we do know, and our knowledge of breast cancer biology, we have come up with some guidelines to follow until we do have the exact scientific answers. We, as physicians and exercise specialists, are actively involved in the pursuit of scientific truth on how to prevent new and recurrent breast cancer. At the Fred Hutchinson Cancer Research Center, and the University of Washington in Seattle, we are conducting several studies to look at the effects of aerobic, weight-training, and stretching exercise programs on some biological markers of breast cancer risk. In this book, we have drawn up some guidelines based on what we have learned from our studies and those of other scientists around the world.

You may want to know when should you start exercising. Is exercise in childhood critical? If you are forty years old and have never exercised or played sports, is it too late to start for reducing breast cancer risk? What kind of exercise is most beneficial? Is it necessary to do strenuous activities such as running, or is moderate exercise such as brisk walking enough? Many women are adding weight training to their exercise routine, to build muscle and burn fat. Will weight training help reduce breast cancer risk? At what age, if ever, can you stop exercising? How many minutes per day should you exercise? Should you exercise every day, or will just some days suffice?

We also do not know much about the additive effects of various means of reducing breast cancer risk. For example, if a woman exercises, avoids alcohol, eats a healthy diet, has her babies at an early age, and takes tamoxifen, how much can she reduce her risk for breast cancer? Tamoxifen works as an antiestrogen. If women reduce their estrogen levels to a minimum after menopause through exercise, fat mass reduction, and diet, could the tamoxifen effect be strengthened?

Throughout this book, we present our guidelines based on the science and biology of breast cancer. We operate on the premise that more is likely better but that each woman needs to decide what exercise program will fit into her life at that stage in her life. We give you hints on how to fit in the time to exercise and how to motivate yourself to start and maintain a program. These hints are based on the science of behavior change, as well as our experience working with thousands of patients, clients, and study participants.

Finally, there are no certainties in science or in life. We do believe that the scientific studies we present have promising results for breast cancer protection. However, reducing risk does not equal eliminating risk. Therefore, as we described in Chapter 4, you should not neglect the other important parts of breast health, including regular mammograms and breast exams by your doctor or health care provider.

Summary

- Obesity, overweight, and lifetime weight gain increase risk for breast cancer after menopause.
- Fat gained in the abdominal area may add the most risk for breast cancer.
- Exercise prevents and controls overweight and obesity and helps to reduce lifetime fat gain.
- Most epidemiological studies have found that women who exercise at higher intensity levels (brisk walking, jogging) for more than three hours per week have about a 30 percent reduced risk of getting breast cancer.
- Some studies found that current exercise was most protective, others found that exercise in teen years was most important, while others found that continued, consistent exercise over the lifetime was most protective.
- Little is known about the association between exercise and breast cancer in racial and ethnic groups other than whites in the United States.
- More research is needed to answer specific questions on the ages women should exercise, how much exercise, what types of exercise, and what intensity exercises are needed to reduce breast cancer risk.
- Research is needed to determine the additive effects of exercise, diet, alcohol avoidance, and use of tamoxifen on breast cancer risk. In other words, how far can a woman reduce her risk if she incorporates several risk reduction measures?

6

Exercise to Reduce Risk— How It Might Work

Exercise has many powerful effects on the body's function throughout the lifespan that could help fight cancer. These anticancer effects could work either at the stage of preventing a cancer from developing or from growing enough to be detectable (in effect preventing or delaying its occurrence), or at the stage of helping the body to fight a cancer that has already grown large enough to be detected and treated. Exercise has various effects on the body's hormonal, reproductive, metabolic, and immunological systems. These various effects could also affect the growth and development of cancer cells. We give you an overview of cancer development in this chapter. We show you how exercise can lower your body's estrogen levels throughout life. We describe the effect of exercise on other hormones that could be related to breast cancer risk. Finally, we present information on the effect of exercise on immune function, a body system that also could be related to breast cancer risk.

The Two Steps in Cancer Development

Researchers believe that the development of cancer is a two-stage process: cancer initiation and cancer promotion. The *initiation* of cancer happens at the level of a single cell's DNA. Some cancer-causing agent, a carcinogen, causes some damage to the DNA that can later lead to abnormal growth. There are many genes involved in the repair of DNA. Your cells are exposed to DNA-damaging agents all the time. One example is sunlight, where ultraviolet radiation causes DNA damage that can eventually lead to melanoma and other skin cancers. Some people have defects in their DNA repair genes, so that even a small amount of DNA damage cannot be fixed, and the cell is left to grow and reproduce erratically and excessively. Besides your own genes, there are substances that can prevent or repair DNA damage. Examples include antioxidant vitamins such as vitamin E and folate. *Promotion* of cancer occurs first at the level of the cell, then at the level of a tumor and its metastases, or spread, to other body sites. There are many potential promoters of breast cancer, including estrogens, androgens (male hormones), insulin, and growth factors. There are also substances that can fight breast cancer promotion. One is the drug tamoxifen, which fights promotion by competing with estrogen and preventing estrogen from entering the breast cell. Your immune system can also fight the promotion of cancer by attacking cancer cells at their origin and when they get into the blood and lymphatic systems.

We believe that exercise could be a cancer promotion fighter, by reducing the amount of blood estrogens and by improving immune function. There is some evidence that estrogen can be a cancer initiator, so that reducing the level of blood estrogen may also fight the initiation of breast cancer.

Exercise Alters Estrogen Production via the Pituitary Gland and Ovaries

Regular exercise, especially vigorous exercise, affects girls' pituitary gland and ovaries with the result of altering and reducing the production of hormones such as estrogen. The balance of these hormones controls when menstrual periods begin, how often they occur, whether they result in a viable egg being released from the ovary, and when they stop at menopause.

A critical amount of female hormones, and a particular pattern of hormone release, is necessary before menarche (the start of menstrual periods) is initiated. Girls can reach this critical hormone level in their early teens or earlier. A reduction in the production of estrogens, or a change in the natural daily variation in estrogen levels, can delay the age at which menstrual periods first start.

The average age of menarche in the United States today is 12.8 years, though many girls get their periods as early as nine or ten. This early age at menarche means that these girls are being exposed to high levels of estrogen starting at a very early age. This early exposure has been found to increase a woman's later risk of getting breast cancer. Girls who are very athletic as children and early teens, however, often do not start their periods until they are sixteen years old or older. This decreases their risk of breast cancer later.

The age of menarche is preceded and paralleled by changes in the breast. During early childhood, all girls have rudimentary breasts, called buds, that lie dormant until enough hormones are produced by the pituitary gland and ovaries to cause a growth in breast tissue. Once the breast growth starts, it continues throughout the teen years. This growth involves development and multiplication of cells lining the milk ducts and of the structures supporting them. Some scientists believe that the breast cells do not finish their rate of rapid growth until a woman's first pregnancy that lasts six months or longer. This effect of pregnancy may explain why women who have had early pregnancies (before age twenty), and who have had several pregnancies, have a decreased risk of developing breast cancer compared to women who have never been pregnant or who had their first pregnancy after age thirty.

Even after a woman is having periods, exercise can have an effect. Women such as competitive athletes who exercise at high levels may go months between periods. When they do have periods, they are likely to be what is called "anovulatory periods." This means that the ovaries are being suppressed enough that an egg is not released, even though some hormones are being produced resulting in menstrual periods. These menstrual changes reflect remarkable underlying hormonal changes in these athletes. The pituitary gland releases smaller amounts of hormones that stimulate the ovary. In response, the ovary makes much less estrogen. This situation is reversible—soon after the level of exercise is reduced, normal ovulation resumes and the woman can become pregnant. (There are situations, however, where it takes some time for an athlete who is having menstrual irregularities to regain normal ovulation and periods.)

The effect of exercise on hormone production can be so strong that some adverse effects can occur in rare cases. In girls and women who exercise at high levels and fail to take in adequate calories, the production of hormones can fall low enough to cause weakening of bones and make them more vulnerable to fractures. Bone weakening is a serious concern of low estrogen levels, especially since it is very difficult to replace bone mass once it has been lost. Clearly there has to be a balance, so that while it may be beneficial to reduce estrogen levels from what most girls and women experience, it is important not to reduce them enough to weaken bones.

Exercise may affect another marker of breast cancer risk. Women whose breasts show particular mammogram patterns with highly dense areas are at increased risk for breast cancer. These dense areas likely represent an increased number and activity of active breast tissues such as ductal systems. Estrogens have been shown to increase these dense areas, and withdrawal of estrogen has been shown to decrease them. Researchers in Norway studied the mammograms of 2,720 women who had been interviewed about their lifestyle and other breast cancer risk factors. They found that women who exercised at high intensity and for long durations had lower amounts of breast density areas. While they could not say that this was caused by the exercise (there may be something else about the exercisers that made their breast densities smaller), it does lend support to a protective effect of exercise on the breast tissues themselves.

ℒ❤   Exercise Lowers Estrogen Production from Fat Cells

As we discuss in Chapter 8, most women's bodies continue to produce small amounts of estrogen after menopause. These estrogens, however, are produced not in the ovaries but in the body fat cells. Fat cells contain a substance called aromatase that converts male hormones such as testosterone into estrogens. Women's bodies make male hormones in their ovaries and in their adrenal glands even after menopause. Even women who have had their ovaries surgically removed continue to produce male hormones in the adrenal glands, although they usually have lower levels of these male hormones compared with women with intact ovaries.

Postmenopausal women who have large amounts of body fat have higher levels of aromatase and produce more estrogens compared with thinner women. Several studies have confirmed this by measuring the amount of estrone and estradiol (the major estrogens in postmenopausal women) in the blood and correlating them to women's weight, body mass index, and body fat distribution. Obese and overweight women have on average estrone and estradiol levels that are almost double those of thin women. The fat cells in breasts contain aromatase, so women with larger, fattier breasts might be expected to make larger amounts of estrogen right in the breast. This has not been proved scientifically, however.

Figure 6.1. Overweight and obese women have high blood estrogen levels.

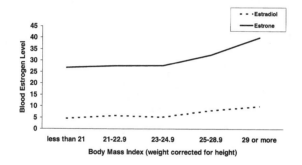

Graph design by Clayton Hibbert.

Figure 6.2. Risk of breast cancer is higher in overweight or obese women.

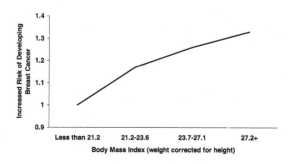

Graph design by Clayton Hibbert.

Regardless of their weight, postmenopausal women who carry more fat around their middle area than around their hips and thighs are likely to have higher levels of estrogen that is unbound to blood proteins, making it more available to act at the level of breast cells. This means that, even if you are not overweight, if you have an "apple" shape rather than a "pear" shape, you should increase your exercise in order to decrease your estrogen levels and thereby decrease the risk to your breasts.

A few studies have looked at the associations between physical activity and levels of blood estrogen after menopause. Dr. Jane Cauley and her colleagues asked 176 postmenopausal women whose average age was fifty-eight about their current physical activity habits and had them wear a device that continuously measured their movements. They divided the women into four categories of usual physical activity and found that women in the highest category of daily physical activity had 15 percent lower levels of estrogen compared with the most sedentary group. When the researchers divided women into four groups according to the movement measuring device, they found that women who measured high on the movement scale had 25 to 30 percent lower estrogen levels compared with the most sedentary women. This association between increased physical activity and decreased estrogen levels was seen in women of all body weights.

Figure 6.3. Exercise is associated with lower estrogen levels in postmenopausal women.

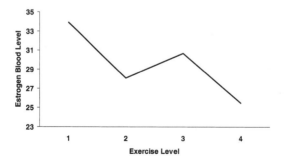

Graph design by Clayton Hibbert.

✍ Exercise Increases Proteins That Bind Estrogen, Rendering It Less Effective

Exercise has beneficial effects on other hormones and body functions, in ways that might reduce risk of breast cancer. Exercise increases a protein called sex hormone binding globulin that carries most of the estrogens and male hormones in the bloodstream. If a woman has more of the protein, it will bind to more of the hormones, thereby leaving less hormone to circulate on its own in the blood. It is the free circulating estrogens or male hormones that are thought to be the most dangerous to the breast cells. Several studies have found that women who have high levels of sex hormone binding globulin have lower risk of getting breast cancer. Most of these studies have also found that high levels of freely circulating male hormones, as well as estrogens, are associated with increased breast cancer risk.

✍ Exercise Reduces Cancer-Promoting Growth Factors

Another hormone that potentially increases the growth rates of cancers, including breast cancer, is insulinlike growth factor, or IGF. IGF stimulates the growth of many body cells and has been shown to increase the growth of cancer cells in the laboratory. Despite its name, it is not an insulin and is not associated with diabetes. At high levels, IGF has been found to be associated with increased risk of breast cancer development. IGF levels are higher in sedentary, overweight women than in lighter, physically active women. IGF levels have been shown to go down when a woman increases her physical activity level. There is a protein that carries IGF in the bloodstream that is increased with physical activity, so that less IGF can circulate freely in the bloodstream in an active woman.

✍ Exercise Lowers Excess Insulin

Exercise lowers insulin and reduces the risk of insulin-resistance, which can lead to adult-onset diabetes. There is some evidence that insulin promotes cancer cell growth in the laboratory, and may do so in the human body as well. Aerobic exercise reduces insulin levels. In diabetics, in fact, exercise alone, if accompanied by as little as three to four pounds of fat loss, can control glucose levels and reduce need for medication.

Exercise Improves Your Immune System

Exercise may result in improvements in the immune system that could protect against cancer. Your body has several defense systems that guard against invasion by foreign substances such as viruses and bacteria. Cancer-causing substances (carcinogens) and cancer cells can also be thought of as foreign substances, if your body recognizes them as something foreign and mounts a fight against them.

The first line of defense against a foreign invader is the barrier system: skin, mucous membranes such as those lining the mouth and nose, and tiny hairs and other systems that actively move invading substances out of the body. For example, research has shown that individuals who drink copious amounts of liquids may have a lower risk of developing bladder cancer—perhaps the continuous flushing of the bladder with liquids helps to propel carcinogens out of the body before they can cause cancer in bladder cells. Individuals who have frequent bowel movements appear to be at reduced risk for developing colon or intestinal cancer. The frequent bowel movements may move carcinogens out and away from the colon, thereby protecting the colon cells. The frequent bowel movements could also protect the breast, if they are also moving estrogens and other breast carcinogens out of your body before they can be reabsorbed into the bloodstream and deposit in your breasts where they can do serious damage. Women who engage in regular aerobic exercise have more frequent bowel movements than women who are sedentary.

Many women's favorite physical activities take them outdoors. This increases sunlight exposure and the sun's vitamin D benefits. Women with increased levels of vitamin D have lower risk for breast cancer, at least in preliminary studies. So exercise could help with the first defense level, the barrier system, in more than one way.

Your body's second level of defense is the cells that rush to where an invader is lurking and surround and kill the foreign object or cell. Other cells circulate in the bloodstream and travel to whatever part of the body is being invaded. Some cells produce substances that are designed to attack a specific agent such as a virus or bacteria. Other cells produce and release cytokines, which are proteins that are toxic to invading foreign matter.

Some immune cells that are particularly strong defenders are called natural killer cells. These cells may be especially protective against cancer. In the laboratory, natural killer cells attack tumor cells and whole tumors with a vengeance. Animals that are deficient in immune cells are more prone to cancer and less able to recover from cancer. There is increasing evidence from research studies that exercise improves the number and strength of natural killer cells and the immune cells' ability to produce cytokines to attack tumor cells.

There are some special circumstances where exercise could have a deleterious temporary effect on the immune system. These seem to happen only with people who are overtraining, such as athletes training at high levels for several hours every day for a competition. Sometimes these athletes push their bodies over the limits in terms of health effects. In addition to the various injuries to muscles, tendons, and bones that you might imagine with overtraining, these athletes can experience an impairment in their immune systems so that they are more prone to colds, flu, and gastrointestinal infections. Luckily, exercise that is less than this competitive level has the opposite effect and causes an improvement in immune function.

Figure 6.4. Regular moderate to vigorous exercise may improve immune function, but excessive training may cause decline in immune function.

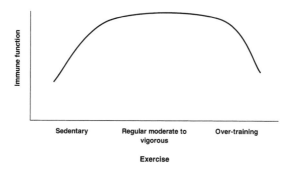

Graph design by Clayton Hibbert.

Summary

Exercise has the following effects, which can explain exercise protection against breast cancer:

- Delays age at which menstruation begins
- Reduces numbers of menstrual cycles with ovulation
- Lengthens menstrual cycles
- Reduces levels of estrogen that is produced by the ovary
- May reduce levels of estrogen that is made in fat cells
- Reduces amount of free estrogen and male hormones in the blood
- May reduce breast densities seen on mammograms
- Reduces levels of insulin and insulinlike growth factor
- Improves immune function, which may affect cancer risk

7

The Role of Nutrition
in Breast Cancer

We believe that exercise and nutrition go hand in hand in effects on health and well-being. The effect of overweight and obesity on increasing risk for breast cancer and on decreasing survival from breast cancer is most likely due to a combination of lack of exercise and poor nutrition. In this chapter, we outline some scientific evidence of nutrition's role in risk of breast cancer. We present information about important new studies of nutrition and breast cancer whose results will be available in a few years. We give you advice about how to improve your nutrition to promote optimal health and to maximize the effectiveness of your exercise program.

You are what you eat. The ability of your body's organs and structures to grow and function depends on what you provide them in nourishment and energy. It is not surprising that diet has been linked to diverse states of health and disease. For centuries it has been recognized that extreme nutritional deficiencies result in disease. Some examples are scurvy from lack of vitamin C, rickets from lack of vitamin D, and anemia from iron deficiency. Observations in this century of some striking associations between dietary substances and risk of certain cancer have raised suspicion of a link between diet and cancer. For example, there appears to be a strong association between a substance called aflatoxin and the development of liver cancer. Aflatoxin is a by-product of certain fungi that grow on grains and other plants such as peanuts. It has toxic effects on the liver and may also cause cancer in the liver. Excess intake of alcoholic beverages has been linked to increased occurrence of cancers of the head and neck. What has been less studied, however, is the effect of more subtle nutritional deficiencies or the effect of certain dietary patterns on risk of cancer.

Excess Intake of Calories

As we described earlier, overweight and obesity are associated with increased risk for developing breast cancer after menopause. Increased body mass in early life may also be a factor in determining later risk of developing breast cancer. An early age at first menstruation increases risk. One factor affecting age at first menstruation is a girl's nutritional and body composition status. Girls who are highly nourished to the extent that they grow tall faster and have early deposits of fat are more likely to have early periods. Some doctors believe that a girl has to reach a critical weight for her age and height in order to start having periods. Girls who have calorie-rich diets and low levels of physical activity are likely to reach this critical weight early. Some researchers believe that the high protein levels of typical North American and European diets promote rapid early growth in childhood, resulting in an early start to puberty and resulting increased risk for breast cancer. The effect of an early age at first menstruation, as described in Chapter 2, may be through increasing estrogen levels during adolescence and early adulthood. There is evidence that the breasts are particularly sensitive to cancer initiation and promotion during the teen and early adult years, especially before a first pregnancy that lasts six months or more.

Later in life, high-calorie diets also promote the deposition of fat stores, especially when the output of energy is low such as in sedentary women. Excess fat stores can raise the levels of insulin, growth factors, and hormones in the blood that can promote the growth of tumors. As we described in Chapter 2, lifetime weight gain was shown in the Nurses' Health Study and other large prospective studies to be associated with increased risk for developing breast cancer after menopause. Although there are some genetic influences on how much fat women gain as they age if their calorie intake exceeds their energy expenditure, virtually all women will gain fat if their calorie intake is too high for their energy needs. To reduce the amount of fat gained during your lifetime, you need to watch your calorie intake. A good way to control overall calorie intake is to increase your intake of vegetables and fruits. If your diet is high in vegetables and fruits, therefore, you will likely take in less of calorie-dense foods like fats and sugars. This will reduce your overall intake of calories and help to avoid gains in fat.

Dietary Fat

If you read newspapers or magazines, or watch TV, you may have seen or heard several conflicting reports about the relationship between dietary fat and risk of breast cancer. The reason you are getting this contradictory information is that scientists have collected inconsistent data. The upshot is that they still do not know what role, if any, dietary fat plays in the development or promotion of breast cancer. Some animal experiments have shown that animals fed high-fat diets get more breast tumors than animals given low-fat diets. Since high-fat diets are usually high in calories, it is difficult to determine if the tumor-promoting effects of the high-fat diets resulted from the fat per se or from the extra calories. Indeed, calorie-restricted diets in experimental animals have been shown to reduce tumor development. Studies comparing rates of breast cancer in countries with high intakes of dietary fat versus countries with low intakes of fat show that the higher the dietary intake of fat in a country, the higher the incidence of breast cancer. However, there are likely many differences in culture and exposure to cancer-causing agents between countries that could explain differences in breast cancer occurrence. Some cross-country differences that are related to breast cancer risk include age at start of puberty, age at first childbirth, number of pregnancies, breast-feeding, body mass, physical activity, use of alcohol, use of oral contraceptives and menopausal hormones, other dietary factors besides dietary fat, and height.

Several large, long-term studies have looked at the role of dietary fat and risk of developing breast cancer. The best of these, where healthy women were queried about their usual dietary patterns and then followed forward in time until some of them developed breast cancer, did not find that dietary fat increased risk of breast cancer. The problem with these studies is that they relied on women reporting what they usually ate. The questionnaires used in these studies do not accurately estimate fat intake in some women, especially in heavier women who may for many reasons underestimate what they are eating. Another problem is that the women in the studies tend to have a rather homogeneous diet. That is, there is a very small range of dietary fat intake, making it difficult to estimate what the risk would be if a woman had a very low-fat diet. A third problem is that these studies collect information about diet in adulthood—none have been able to assess the role of dietary patterns in childhood and teen years and later development of breast cancer. It may be that since the young breast is the most vulnerable to cancer initiation and early promotion, dietary patterns early in life are more important than adult dietary patterns.

There is some discrepancy about whether all fats could be related to increased risk for breast cancer. Some animal experiments suggest that all fats could increase tumor development, while others point to polyunsaturated fats (which are derived from plant sources) as the most dangerous. Some researchers have suggested that monounsaturated fats, which are present in high quantities in olive and canola oils, may not increase risk for breast cancer. This could explain the lower incidence of breast cancer in countries such as Italy and Greece with high intake of olive oil. Alternatively, there may be some special properties of olive oil such as vitamin content that might protect against breast cancer.

That dietary fat might have direct effects on the breast in humans is supported by a study done in Canada by Dr. Norman Boyd and his colleagues. They recruited women with increased risk for breast cancer by virtue of having high levels of density patterns on their mammograms. Density patterns on mammograms may reflect underlying estrogen activity in the breast and likely represents high levels of breast cell growth and proliferation. In Dr. Boyd's study, the women were randomly assigned to a very low-fat diet or to their usual diet. After two years of follow-up, women eating the very low-fat diet had a significant reduction in the amount of breast density. This study is significant in that it indicates that a low-fat diet can produce biological effects in the breast, and that it can do so in a relatively short period of time. Furthermore, it points out that breast density revealed on mammograms could serve as a tool for following individual women's progress in their efforts at reducing their risk of breast cancer.

The only way to answer the question, finally, of whether high intakes of dietary fat increase breast cancer risk is to conduct a randomized clinical trial of a dietary fat pattern and risk of breast cancer development in women. The Women's Health Initiative is a sixteen-year study funded by the National Institutes of Health to look at the effect of diet, hormone therapy, and calcium and vitamin D on various diseases that affect women after menopause. Coordinated by the Fred Hutchinson Cancer Research Center, the study has recruited more than 160,000 women age fifty to seventy-nine into forty clinical centers across the United States. Dr. Ross Prentice and Dr. Maureen Henderson and their colleagues at Hutchinson and across the country did much of the preliminary work that led to the recognition of the need for a large-scale, long-term clinical trial of a low-fat dietary pattern effect on breast cancer incidence. This early work included complex statistical analyses of geographic correlations between dietary fat intake and breast cancer rates across the country, as well as studies to show that given the right knowledge and tools, women are very successful at adopting a low-fat dietary pattern and at maintaining the new eating habits over several years.

In the Women's Health Initiative dietary study, more than 48,000 women who were currently following a high-fat diet were assigned by chance to adopt either a very low-fat diet or to retain their current diet. (The key part of this study is this assignment by chance, which is called randomization. Randomization assures that the things that might be different about women who choose on their own to follow a low-fat diet are controlled for. Randomization minimizes the chance of a study producing biased results.) The diet consists of reducing fat to 20 percent or less of total calorie intake, increasing servings of fruits/vegetable to five per day, and increasing servings of grains (bread, pasta, etc.) to six per day. All of the women are being followed for at least eight to twelve years to look at the effect of the diet on risk of breast cancer and other diseases. The results of the Women's Health Initiative will not be known until about 2005.

The Canadian study of Dr. Boyd and colleagues is examining the impact of a low-fat eating pattern on breast cancer occurrence in 9,500 women with breast densities on their mammograms and who are therefore at increased risk for developing breast cancer.

Many women and scientists are interested in knowing whether dietary fat can influence prognosis for women with breast cancer. As we describe in Chapter 10, women who are overweight or obese, or who gain weight after breast cancer diagnosis, have poorer survival compared with thinner women. The Women's Intervention Nutrition Study is looking at the effect of a very low-fat diet on breast cancer prognosis and survival. In this study, 2,500 women with breast cancer are being recruited by more than fifty clinics across the United States. The patients are randomized to either a very low-fat diet or to their current diet. With the very low-fat diet, patients are asked to decrease their intake of fat to fifteen percent or less of their total daily calories. The results of this study will also not be known for several years. The Women's Healthy Eating and Lifestyle Study is testing a plant-based diet high in vegetables and fruit in about 3,000 breast cancer patients, to look at diet's effect on breast cancer recurrence.

✍ Vitamins and Minerals

The insight that the rates of breast cancer vary so much by country has led some scientists to focus on fruits and vegetables, and their content of vitamins and minerals, as the key links between diet and risk of breast cancer. Some vitamins and minerals contain substances called antioxidants, which work to repair the cell's DNA after it has been damaged by environmental causes such as X rays, sunlight, and chemicals. Some vitamins can also regulate the rate of growth of breast cells. Some epidemiological studies have found that women with diets high in vitamins A (including retinol and beta-carotene), C, D, or E had decreased risk for getting breast cancer. There are substances on breast cells that can bind to vitamin D, which indicates that vitamin D may play a role in the biology of breast cells.

Clinical trials are underway to test the effects of some of these vitamins by randomly giving women either vitamin or placebo pills and following them to observe which group develops more breast cancers. The Women's Health Initiative is testing the effect of a pill that combines calcium and vitamin D on the risk of various diseases including breast cancer. The Women's Health Study, a randomized clinical trial in 40,000 United States female health professionals, is testing the effect of vitamins E and D on the development of breast cancer among other disease outcomes. There have also been several clinical trials of beta-carotene and retinol that may provide future data on the effects of these vitamins on breast cancer incidence.

In animal experiments, supplementation with selenium inhibited breast cancer development, even after the animals were treated with potent cancer-causing chemicals. Selenium may prevent cancer by working as an antioxidant, by improving immune function, by suppressing excess breast cell growth, or by altering the metabolism of cancer-causing substances. Studies in women have not yielded consistent information about the effect of selenium on breast cancer risk. This may be because selenium intake is difficult to measure either by asking women about their diets or by measuring levels in blood. Selenium is present in the soil to differing degrees in different geographical areas; dietary intake depends on where produce was grown. A clinical trial in which women and men were randomly assigned to selenium or placebo pills showed some promise of selenium in reducing risk of some cancers. The National Cancer Institute is conducting further studies of this mineral as a possible prevention agent against several cancers.

A few epidemiologic studies have found that women with high intakes of calcium have lower risk for breast cancer, but many studies have found no effect of calcium. One problem is that in previous years, women who had high intakes of calcium-containing foods also took in more fat and calories than women with low-calcium diets. The role of calcium in breast cancer remains unclear.

Protein

There is much less information about the association between dietary protein and breast cancer risk. In animal studies, diets that are low in protein result in delayed sexual maturity, reduced body growth rates, and decreased incidence of breast tumors. There have been few studies in humans, and results have been mixed. While a couple of studies indicated that women with high daily protein intakes had increased risk for breast cancer, other studies found no association between protein and risk. Since there is so little information on this nutrient, we do not make any specific recommendations about limiting protein intake to reduce breast cancer risk. However, if you are trying to reduce your calorie and fat intake, you are likely not eating much high-fat protein such as red meat. By reducing your intake of calories and fat, and increasing your intake of fruits and vegetables, you will naturally lower your intake of protein if you currently have a high intake of animal proteins. Most women need at least 50 grams of protein each day, however. Teenage, pregnant, and nursing women need at least 60–75 grams per day. Good low-fat, low-calorie sources of protein include soy, legumes (beans), fish, and poultry. Eggs, although high in cholesterol, are also an excellent source of protein.

Vegetarian Diets

If you follow a vegetarian diet, be sure to read labels and pay attention to the fat content of your food. A vegetarian diet does not guarantee a low-fat diet. Soy products such as tofu can contain a large amount of fat. Creamy pasta sauces can be very high in fat and calories. Vegetarians may also tend to eat more cheese as a protein, which is usually high in fat. A *vegan* diet excludes dairy products so is usually lower in fat content. If you are having trouble getting enough low-fat protein in your vegetarian or vegan diet, try adding a protein supplement. Protein supplements or powders are fat free and can be mixed with cow, soy, or rice milk. Protein supplements are not meal substitutes but are a way to maintain appropriate amounts of protein in your diet. Be sure to limit sweets and baked goods such as cookies, cakes, croissants, and muffins because they usually contain high amounts of fat.

Vegetarian diets can also be deficient in some minerals and vitamins that are found only in meats. If you eat no meat or eggs, you may not be getting enough vitamin B^{12}, zinc, or iron. These vitamins are very important for immune system and other body functions. Iron is very important for menstruating, pregnant, and breast-feeding women. If you do not eat dairy products, your calcium intake may be deficient. You should get at least 1,200 milligrams of calcium each day (1,500 milligrams if you are postmenopausal). The safest thing is to take a daily mineral and vitamin supplement that includes these vitamins and minerals, and separate calcium supplements to get your daily minimum requirement.

Using Nutrition to Enhance Exercise Performance

Athletes have known for many years that what they eat affects how well they can compete and perform. Nutrition needs for athletic performance are directly related to the type, amount, and intensity of exercise you do. In general, low-fat, high-carbohydrate calories are best when fueling any exercise. The amount of calories you need to fuel your workouts depends on the amount and intensity of exercise you do. If you exercise three hours a week, your caloric demand is lower than if you exercise six hours a week. You need a different amount of calories for maintaining your weight through exercise than for using exercise to lose weight. Endurance exercise such as long-distance running, where you are exercising for more than an hour, requires more calories than short jogging sessions.

The number of calories you should eat on any given day depends on three factors. The first factor is your metabolic "set point," which is determined by genetics, your gender, and your body size. Your set point is the number of calories you need to keep basic metabolic functions operating properly to sustain life. This means how many calories you need to keep your hair growing, eyelids blinking, heart pumping, lungs breathing, etc. The second factor is the number of calories you need for your activities of daily life. You need more calories if you do physical labor most of the day than if you sit most of the day. The third factor is your exercise program. These are the calories you expend when you exercise. Heather Nakamura, a nutrition and exercise expert who works with Dr. McTiernan's studies in Seattle, has developed an example of the calorie contents of some foods and the amount of exercise needed to burn that amount of calories (see Table 7.1).

Table 7.1. Amount of Exercise Required for a 154-Pound Woman to Burn Off Calories in Specific Foods

FOOD	CALORIES	ACTIVITY	TIME REQUIRED (MINUTES)
Peanuts, 1 cup	840	Walking 3 mph	227
Fast-food chicken, two-piece dinner	720	Bicycling	180
Trail mix, 1 cup	700	Walking 4 mph	127
Fast-food chicken sandwich	700	Walking 4 mph	127
Milkshake, large	640	Walking 3 mph	173
Fast-food hamburger, large	500	Walking 3 mph	135

FOOD	CALORIES	ACTIVITY	TIME REQUIRED (MINUTES)
Raisins, 1 cup	440	Walking 4 mph	80
Ice cream, 1 cup	350	Walking 3 mph	95
Bagel	340	Bicycling	85
Candy bar, 2.2 ounces	280	Bicycling	70
Chocolate cake, slice	250	Walking 3 mph	68
Brownie, 3" x 3"	200	Walking 4 mph	36
Pepperoni pizza, slice	120	Bicycling	30

Carbohydrates provide immediate energy for exercise. Some athletes do what is called "carbo loading." This involves eating larger quantities than usual of high-carbohydrate foods for a few days prior to a heavy workout or competition. This extra carbohydrate is "loaded" into the muscles to help fuel up for the increased demand on the body during heavy training and competition. Long-distance bicyclists sometimes find that they need to eat energy-dense foods frequently while they are biking. Nutrient bars are simply high-calorie foods that can help some athletes keep up their energy needs. Women who are exercising at less intense levels and not using up as many calories during their workout, however, should be sure to check the calorie and nutrient content of these nutrient bars before making them a regular part of their diet.

Carbohydrates fuel your workouts, but proteins are the building blocks of every cell in your body. Many of your body's cells need to be constantly replaced. Without adequate protein in your diet, you could become more fatigued during your workouts and throughout your activities of daily living. The best diet includes a balance of adequate protein and carbohydrate that gives you maximum energy for your workouts and the rest of your activities.

When you exercise, you lose fluid, primarily through sweating. If you have less energy during workouts or training, it may be due to lack of hydration rather than lack of calories. Aerobic exercise is dependent on efficient metabolic pathways and a strong muscle system. Muscle continuity is improved with water intake by enhancing the muscle's ability to contract and swell. The best way to tell if you are drinking enough water is by your urine. When you are properly hydrated, your urine should be a pale yellow. If it is dark yellow, you need to drink more water. Other fluids such as sport drinks help some women keep up their electrolytes and calories when exercising. Electrolyes are chemicals such as sodium and potassium that keep proper balance in your cells and body fluid.

Exercising at high levels, as with training, can cause stress at the level of some cells. This is called oxidative stress. Some scientists believe that some vitamins and minerals, the antioxidants, can help to fight this type of stress to your body. Be sure to take at least a multivitamin that contains the antioxidant vitamins and minerals (beta-carotene, selenium, vitamins A, C, and E) every day if you are in training.

Changing Diet Behaviors

Eating is more than just nourishment. Eating has many emotional and cultural meanings to people. If you make a commitment to eat a healthier diet, you need to understand what motivates you to eat certain things. Then you need to learn some tools to help you change your eating behavior.

You learned many of your food preferences and dislikes as a child from your family and friends. You may have developed warm associations with some foods, and these may be for you what we call "comfort foods." These could be foods that were served at special family events such as holiday meals. They could be certain foods that were routinely served at family meals. They could be foods your parents gave you as treats or rewards. Or you may have developed preferences for some foods that satisfy an urge for you or that just make you feel better.

There could be physiological reasons for your preferences for certain comfort foods. Foods that are high in carbohydrates raise your brain levels of serotonin, which is a chemical that provides a feeling of well-being and relaxation. Serotonin is what causes that sleepy feeling you may get after eating a big pasta meal. Foods that are high in fat provide a full sensation that leaves you feeling satisfied for several hours after you eat. For many people, sweets provide pleasurable feelings and associations. Chocolate is the ultimate comfort food for many people, especially women. It is high in carbohydrates from sugar, high in fat, and sweet in flavor, so that it provides several of the comforting sensations we have been talking about. In addition, chocolate includes chemicals that provide direct stimulation of the brain's pleasure and arousal centers. So how can you overcome your urges for comfort foods? Many nutritionists suggest that you not completely deny yourself the foods that you crave and that provide comfort. Rather, they say to limit the quantities of these foods if they are high in calories, fat, or sugar. Fill up on low-calorie foods first, then allow yourself a few bites of the comfort food. If you are sufficiently full from the low-calorie foods, then you will get the same comforting feelings from just a few bites.

Much of your dietary pattern as an adult is a result of what you were taught as a child. The recipes and food preparation techniques you know were what your parents (usually mother) taught you. The amount of food you prefer to eat was also likely taught to you as a child. Many of these traditional family eating patterns were passed down from generations back, when food variety was rare and energy expenditure was high. Our parents and grandparents expended much more energy in their home and work lives. Thus, they needed to take in more food calories to match the calories they burned each day. They developed recipes and food patterns that would provide these calories. Unless they were wealthy, they also did not have access to expensive cuts of meat or to fresh vegetables and fruits. Foods such as stews with thick fatty gravies, potatoes mashed with milk and butter, cakes and pies, were the result.

The recent dramatic changes in our modern home and lives resulted in much less energy needed to live and work. As a result, adults and children are fatter today than in previous generations. If you want to prevent weight gain as you age, you are going to have to develop new food traditions for yourself and your family. You probably already eat some meals that are different from what your parents provided. However, the modern trend toward more fast food and frozen meals does not provide the adjustment downward in calories that you are going to need to balance your calorie intake with your energy output.

Reducing Your Daily Calorie Intake

One of the marvelous things about our modern life is that we have available more low-calorie foods than we ever did in the past. Fresh vegetables and fruits are available year-round. You can markedly reduce your daily calorie intake just by loading up on vegetables and fruits. Many of the successful commercial weight control programs include high intake of vegetables and fruits as part of their guidelines. In addition to being low in calories and fat, these foods provide more bulk, fiber, and water so that they fill you up faster, making you less likely to reach for the more calorie-dense foods. So the first step in losing weight or in controlling weight gain should be to increase your intake of vegetables and fruits. You can eat as many as you want, although if you are trying to lose weight you may want to limit your intake of the more calorie-rich vegetables and fruits such as potatoes, avocados, corn, cherries, bananas, and peas. Don't eliminate these—just don't use them to fill you up. Table 7.2 presents a list of low-calorie vegetables and fruits.

Table 7.2. Low-Calorie Vegetables and Fruits

VEGETABLES	FRUITS
Asparagus	Apples
Beets	Apricots
Broccoli	Berries, all types
Cabbage	Grapefruit
Carrots	Grapes
Celery	Kiwi
Cucumbers	Melon
Lettuce	Nectarines
Mushrooms	Oranges
Peppers	Peaches
Summer squash	Pears
Tomatoes	Pineapple
Turnips	Plums
Zucchini	Tangerines

Another way to reduce your calorie intake is to increase your water intake. Water helps to fill you up, so that you have less urge to eat higher-calorie foods. In addition, water is necessary for food metabolism, so that if you drink more water you will burn more of the calories you take in. Finally, water makes you feel better. Many women do not drink enough water and go through their day in a dehydrated state. Being dehydrated can make you feel tired or light-headed and can produce problems with concentration and other brain function. Many women overeat in an effort to get the fluids they need; that is, they mistake their body's thirst signals as hunger signals. When you are feeling hungry, first try drinking a couple of glasses of water before eating food. This is a good habit to help you discover when you are actually thirsty rather than hungry. Your weight control program will include increased exercise, which will further increase your need for water. You should drink at least twelve 8-ounce glasses of water or noncaffeinated fluids (such as juice or milk) each day. (This recommendation may need to be adapted to your own body size and activity level. Be aware of the calorie content of juice and milk if you drink a lot of these.) Caffeine drinks do not count toward your fluid requirement. In fact, caffeine is a weak diuretic, which causes you to pass more urine, resulting in greater dehydration. Therefore, a glass of water may be all that you need to feel less tired instead of another cup of coffee. You may find that you can drink more water if you keep a sport bottle of water around you, where you exercise, in your car, in your office. If you feel bloated after drinking fluids, or feel that water "is going right through you," it may be a sign that you are drinking too much water. More likely, though, it is a sign that your fluid regulators are out of balance and that your body is unable to absorb the sudden flood of water into your system. In this case, drinking smaller amounts of water throughout the day will gradually bring your intake and output of fluid into balance.

There are other ways of keeping track of your food intake, if counting calories is frustrating and difficult for you. You might find it simpler to count protein grams instead of calories. You can be sure you eat the necessary 50 grams of protein each day and then fill the rest of your diet up with low-fat, high-fiber foods. You may find that when you are exercising, the number of calories you eat to maintain health is less important than what types of foods you eat to reach your goals.

Keeping a Food Diary

Many research studies have shown that women who write down what they eat lose weight more successfully than women who do not record their dietary intake. Writing down what you eat accomplishes several things. First, it forces you to take a good look at what you are eating all through the day. Second, since you need to record the amount of food you eat, it gives you an idea of your portion sizes—how much of each food you are eating. Third, it gives you information about your dietary patterns, whether you are eating the same thing each day or whether you have a varied diet. It forces you to read the labels on prepared foods so that you know their contents. Finally, it gives you the opportunity to calculate your total intake of calories and fat. You can write down what you eat in your daily calendar journal, or buy a log book specially designed to record food intake.

Diet Supplement Drinks and Meals

Some diet physicians and researchers recommend prepared diet supplement drinks and foods as a way to reduce calories. These supplements contain balanced amounts and proportions of calories, protein, carbohydrates, vitamins, and minerals. If you like to have a meal on the run, these supplement drinks may work for you. However, they may not provide all of the nutritional components that you would get with a healthy balance diet. Most of these do not supply enough calories for one meal, which can cause some women to eat more of other foods such as sweets a few hours after one of these "meals." Therefore we do not recommend that you use these supplements for more than one meal per day.

"Fad" or Extreme Diets

Every year, many new diets come onto the market, each promising to be the answer to every overweight person's dreams. The truth is that *any* diet that lowers total calorie intake results in short-term weight loss. The problem is that more than 80 percent of people who lose weight on a diet eventually regain the weight within a year. Extreme diets, whether they are popular diets or ones that people choose on their own, can be dangerous to your health. If you don't get all of the necessary daily vitamins and minerals, you could be putting yourself at greater risk for cancer than if you stayed overweight, and you could put yourself at serious risk for other health problems. If you don't eat enough protein, you can put your body's internal organs and muscles at risk. If you don't eat enough carbohydrates, your body chemistry can change so that you have higher than normal levels of blood acids that over time can damage your body. If your fat intake is too low, you have an increased risk of developing serious diseases such as gallstones and pancreatitis. See our nutrition recommendations for helping you to reduce excess body fat slowly and keep it off.

Limitations of Current Knowledge

One of the challenges with researching the effects of what people eat on their risk of cancer is that there are so many different foods eaten, in different amounts, and with different preparations. Researchers who find an association between particular nutrients and cancer risk can never be sure if the effect is from one type of nutrient, for example one type of vegetable, or the effect is from the whole dietary pattern. For example, women who eat copious amounts of tomatoes may have lower risk of some cancers. However, women who eat a diet high in tomatoes also typically eat many other vegetables, may eat more than the average amount of pasta (with tomato sauce), and may cook all of their vegetables in olive oil. A finding of protection from tomatoes may just be a reflection of the whole dietary pattern. Similarly, the low risk associated by some researchers with a "Mediterranean" diet may be related to something else about the countries where the diet is consumed. For example, the Mediterranean countries are warm and sunny, and people living there have plenty of sun exposure, leading to higher blood vitamin D levels. Vitamin D has some anticancer properties, so this could explain the low breast cancer risk in the Mediterranean countries.

Recommendations

Until scientists have definitive proof of the associations between diet and breast cancer, it seems prudent to follow the National Cancer Institute guidelines for reducing risks of various cancers:

- Limit intake of fats and oils to less than 30 percent of daily calories.
- Limit intake of salt-preserved foods.
- Minimize consumption of smoked foods.

- Include a variety of fruits and vegetables in the daily diet.
- Increase fiber intake to 20–30 grams per day.

Summary

- Dietary habits or patterns are in some way very likely related to risk of breast cancer.
- Excess intake of calories, as it relates to excess weight gain in childhood, adolescence, and adulthood, may be a key part of the relationship between diet and breast cancer risk.
- Too many calories in relation to energy needs in childhood and adolescence can result in early start of menstrual periods, which increases breast cancer risk.
- Too many calories in relation to energy needs in adulthood can result in a gain in fat over the years, which increases breast cancer risk.
- A high-fat diet can raise your body's levels of estrogens. High levels of estrogens can initiate and promote breast cancer growth.
- A low-fat dietary pattern can improve mammogram patterns to ones associated with reduced risk for breast cancer.
- The "Mediterranean" diet, with its increased emphasis on vegetables and carbohydrates, and decreased emphasis on protein and fats, may be protective. One hypothesis is that olive oil, the most commonly used fat in Mediterranean countries, could have special properties such that it does not increase breast cancer risk.
- Some vitamins could reduce risk for breast cancer by their antioxidant properties, acting to prevent or repair damage to the breast cell's DNA.
- In order to adopt a healthy eating pattern you should: (1) identify and record what you currently eat; (2) increase your intake of vegetables and fruits to reduce dietary sugars, carbohydrates, and fats; (3) not deny yourself high-calorie comfort foods—rather, limit the amount that you eat; (4) develop

new food traditions for yourself, family, and friends that fit with your modern lifestyle and your health needs; and (5) balance your energy intake with your energy output.

- The National Cancer Institute currently recommends a diet that contains no more than 30 percent of calories from fat and five or more servings a day of fruits and vegetables, to help control risk for various cancers. Whether a low-fat dietary pattern will reduce risk for new or recurrent breast cancer will not be known until results are available from the Women's Health Initiative and the Women's Intervention Nutrition Study.

8

The Role of Hormones
in Breast Cancer

Breast cancer is hormone related. This means that in some way, hormones are involved in the development of breast cancer. In this chapter, we introduce the biology of estrogen as it relates to the breast and breast cancer. We present estrogen's role in a girl's development and maturation. We describe the role of estrogen in reproduction. We give information about estrogen's effects on various body systems including the heart, blood vessels, bones, brain, and gallbladder. We present information about other hormones, including progesterone and testosterone, and their potential role in breast cancer.

Many breast cancers grow under the influence of estrogen and regress when estrogen is withdrawn or blocked from acting. In the laboratory, many breast cancer cells grow at a high rate if estrogen is added to the cells. The effect of estrogen is right at the level of the gene—estrogen binds to a protein in the nucleus of the cell, migrates to the genes on the cell's DNA, and stimulates them to produce proteins. When these genes are activated, they produce factors that stimulate growth in cells. They can also stimulate proto-oncogenes, which are genes involved in the development of cancers. In women with breast cancer, removal of all sources of estrogen causes a slowdown in growth of the cancer. In the past, this was accomplished through removing the ovaries and the adrenal glands. Today, this is accomplished by giving drugs, such as tamoxifen, that block estrogen.

Hormones are also important in the treatment of breast cancer. The most important hormone in breast cancer is estrogen, but other hormones such as androgens ("male" hormones) and those related to metabolism and growth are also involved in the growth and development of breast cancer. This chapter tells how estrogens and androgens are made, what effects they have on normal sexual development and reproduction in women, and how they are related to breast cancer.

What Is Estrogen?

Estrogen refers to a particular chemical group of substances that exert control of function of certain kinds of cells. Several estrogens are important in human females. Estradiol is the estrogen that is present in the highest concentration in young women and has the strongest biological activity. Estrone is the second most important estrogen in women. It is produced in smaller amounts in young women. After menopause, however, estrone becomes the dominant estrogen. (A description of how estrogen is produced after menopause follows later in this chapter.) There are other estrogens produced in the body, but in smaller concentrations. Their significance is largely unknown. Estrogens are metabolized in the liver into many other compounds. Some of these compounds are more active than others. Some scientists believe that the relative fractions of different estrogen metabolites are important in breast cancer development. How women's bodies metabolize estrogens, and how different types of metabolites are produced, is under both genetic and environmental control. Environmental factors that can affect what kinds of metabolites are produced include diet, smoking, and alcohol. Women whose diets are high in some vegetables such as broccoli may have a more favorable pattern of estrogen metabolites. There has not been much strong research in this area, however. Most studies have been small and preliminary in nature, and the laboratory evaluation of metabolites is technically quite difficult.

How Estrogen Travels Around Your Body

Estrogen travels in the bloodstream hooked to a protein called sex hormone binding globulin. Some estrogen is bound to a different protein, albumin. This portion of estrogen that is linked to a protein is called "bound" estrogen, and the estrogen that circulates in blood on its own is called "free" estrogen. Some scientists believe that only the "free" hormone can have an effect on cells, although others believe that any estrogen, whether bound or free, can exert actions on cells. There are several things that affect how much hormone is bound and how much is free. Genetics play a role, as the production of binding proteins is somewhat under genetic control. Sex hormone binding globulin is affected by several other factors, including obesity, diet, physical activity, liver function, use of external hormones such as birth control pills or hormone replacement, and other hormones such as growth hormones. Women who are obese, who have large amounts of fat in their middle (as opposed to hips and thighs), and who are sedentary tend to have lower amounts of sex hormone binding globulin. This translates into higher amounts of free, active estrogen throughout life.

How Estrogen Works in the Cell

Estrogen exerts its action in cells directly in the nucleus. Estrogen gets right into the center of the cell's operation, as it influences the function of the cell's DNA. There are substances in the wall of the nucleus, called estrogen receptors, that allow estrogen into the nucleus. Without these receptors, it is believed, estrogen cannot exert its actions in the cell. There are estrogen receptors in many parts of the body, including the breast, uterus, vagina, urethra, brain, bone, skin, vascular system, and intestine. This explains some of the symptoms women feel when they have excess amounts of estrogen (as in pregnancy) or when they have reduced amount of estrogen (as in menopause). Excessive estrogen can cause breast soreness, increased or irregular vaginal bleeding, increased body hair production, and infertility. Decreased estrogen levels, such as in menopause, can cause symptoms such as hot flashes, night sweats, palpitations, decrease in concentration, vaginal and urethral dryness, and skin dryness.

Production of Estrogen

Estrogens can be produced in several areas of the body. In girls and premenopausal women, the ovaries produce the vast majority of estrogen. Estrogen is produced in other parts of the body, however. Some cells can convert androgen into estrogen with an enzyme called aromatase. Aromatase has been found in cells in fat stores, and in muscle, liver, and brain cells. In overweight and obese women, the greatest amount of activity of aromatase is seen in fat. Obese women may produce significant amount of estrogen in fat tissue. In premenopausal women, this excess production of estrogen may interfere with fertility, as the precise release of estrogen needed for fertility gets interrupted with the extra estrogen. In postmenopausal obese or overweight women, fat tissue may produce enough estrogen to cause vaginal bleeding. This estrogen produced after menopause is known to increase risk for breast cancer in women producing high amounts, compared with women producing little estrogen. The estrogen produced after menopause may have some benefits, such as on bone by preventing osteoporosis. Women who are overweight or obese, or who are sedentary, produce more estrogen after menopause compared with lighter, active women. Diet also affects estrogen production. Research has shown that premenopausal and postmenopausal women who are assigned by chance to eat a low-fat or a high-fiber diet produce less estrogen. Alcohol, on the other hand, increases estrogen levels since it affects the liver, where estrogen is metabolized. Soy and some other vegetable products can have estrogen effects in the body. In premenopausal women, soy may compete with natural estrogen to reduce the amount of estrogen affecting cells. In postmenopausal women, conversely, soy may act as an estrogen in its own right and produce estrogenic effects. The effects of diet, alcohol, and soy are described more in Chapters 2 and 7.

Estrogen and Development

Females are first exposed to estrogens when they are fetuses. Pregnant women produce very large amounts of estrogen, and some of this estrogen reaches the developing fetus. Some newborn babies even have little breasts and some breast fluid. This breast fluid, called "witches' milk" in traditional language, disappears soon after birth as the source of estrogen (mom's uterus) is withdrawn. After birth, very little estrogen is produced until the girl has grown enough to have reached a critical level of height and weight. This critical level varies from girl to girl and may be under some genetic influence. A few years before the start of menstrual periods, girls are going through physical changes caused by the increased production of estrogen. Estrogen causes girls' tiny ovaries to enlarge and begin to function as reproductive organs. Estrogen causes the tiny breast "buds" to develop into breast ducts and sacs where milk will eventually be produced and released. Estrogen is responsible for the development of the vagina from a small pouch into a longer, lubricated organ and enlargement of the clitoris, in preparation for adult sexual activity. Estrogen influences how body fat is distributed, resulting in fat depositing primarily in the breasts, hips, buttocks, and thighs. Estrogen affects bone development too. At about the time that a girl begins to menstruate, the rate of bone growth slows considerably. Most girls have a large growth spurt just before menstrual periods start, and stop growing within one to two years after their menstrual periods start. Finally, the right amount of estrogen and the right pattern to its release into the bloodstream are critical in establishing regular periods with the release of an egg. Some girls produce an excess of estrogen, compared with the amount of another female hormone—progesterone—early in their teen years. This can result in heavy and prolonged menstrual bleeding. Doctors often treat this by giving progesterone (birth control) pills.

Estrogen and Reproduction

Estrogen is a key component of reproduction. It keeps the uterus and ovaries ready for pregnancy. During pregnancy, estrogen works with other hormones to produce enlarged functional breasts, changes in the uterine lining making it more hospitable for the developing fetus, and growth and development of the placenta and its blood flow that nourishes the growing fetus. Estrogens also regulate the production in pregnancy of other hormones such as progesterone and cortisol. Estrogens are responsible for that familiar nausea of pregnancy as excess levels of estrogens are irritating to the stomach lining. In concert with several other hormones, estrogen primes the pregnant breast to be ready for lactation (milk production) after childbirth.

Estrogen and the Female Breast

Estrogen has important effects on the female breast. Under the influence of estrogen and other sex hormones, a girl's tiny breast buds grow and develop into glands that will eventually be able to produce milk after a pregnancy. The buds grow into structures called ducts and lobules. The lobules are where the milk is produced. The ducts are the passageways through which the milk is pulled out to the nipples when a baby suckles. There are many lobules and ducts in the breast, and they appear to be arranged into several independent systems, although the exact architecture of the breast is not clearly known. Surrounding the lobules and ducts is what is called the stromal tissue, or supporting structures. The stromal tissue keeps the glandular structures from falling into each other. The stromal tissue also has cells that provide other functions, including cells that make hormones such as estrogen. Surrounding the stromal tissue are deposits of fat. The amount of fat in the breast is what usually determines breast size. The amount of breast fat, in turn, is influenced by genetics, by how much fat a woman has overall, by age, and by her pregnancy and breast-feeding history. Interspersed among all of these structures in the breast are networks of blood vessels, lymph nodes and lymph vessels, and nerves. The amount of ducts, lobules, and stromal tissue relative to the amount of fat determines the density of the breast. Many studies have shown that women with dense breasts, that is, who have a large amount of ducts, lobules, and stromal tissue, have an increased risk of developing breast cancer. We don't know why having dense breasts increases risk. For now, we just use it as a marker of increased risk. Diet, exercise, and some medications can decrease breast density and therefore might be expected to affect risk of getting breast cancer.

Estrogen also affects the sensations a woman experiences in her breasts. Women with high blood estrogen levels often experience pain and tenderness in their nipples and in the rest of the breasts. Many women notice that during pregnancy they have very tender breasts—this symptom is likely due to the very large quantities of estrogen and other sex hormones that are produced during pregnancy. Women who have reached menopause, and therefore make little estrogen on their own, often develop tender or painful breasts if they take estrogen replacement therapy. This symptom may be exacerbated if they take progesterone as well as estrogen.

Estrogen Effects on the Heart and Blood Vessels

Estrogen has very potent effects on other parts of the body as well. Estrogen lowers levels of total and LDL cholesterol (so-called bad cholesterol) and raises HDL cholesterol (the good cholesterol). Estrogen also decreases the stiffness of arteries and improves blood flow through these blood vessels. Estrogen has adverse effects on the circulation, however, by increasing blood's ability to clot. When clotting occurs in the arteries supplying the heart, a heart attack can result. When clotting occurs in veins, the result can be blood clots in the legs (deep vein thrombosis) or in the lungs (pulmonary embolism). The net effect on the heart and other parts of the circulation is unknown. The Heart Estrogen/Progestin Replacement Study (HERS) randomly assigned 2,763 women who already had heart disease to get either hormone replacement (estrogen plus progesterone) or placebo. After following the women for an average of four years, they found that women who received the hormone replacement therapy pills had more heart attacks in the first year on the study compared with women who were given placebo. After the first year, there were fewer heart attacks in the women taking hormone replacement therapy. Some physicians are now saying that women who already have heart disease should not be prescribed hormone therapy. The effect of hormone replacement on heart disease in healthy women is being tested in more than 27,000 women in the Women's Health Initiative Hormone Replacement Clinical Trial. The results of that study, however, won't be known until at least 2005.

Estrogen and the Brain

Estrogen may have beneficial effects on mental functioning. There are estrogen receptors in the brain, meaning that the estrogen that circulates in blood can stick to brain cells and perform its actions on those cells. Some women find that they have problems with concentration and memory as they go through menopause and that these symptoms are relieved with hormone replacement therapy. The effects of estrogen on cognition, or thinking ability, are being tested in a study in some of the Women's Health Initiative participants.

Estrogen Effects on Bones

Estrogen strengthens bones, preventing osteoporosis or thinning of the bones. Early in menopause, when estrogen levels are declining, women experience a rapid loss of bone mass, up to 1 percent of their mass each year. This rate of bone loss is greatest early in menopause and levels off in older ages. The overall effect, however, is a gradual, relentless decline in bone thickness and strength. Thin bones break more easily. An older woman with osteoporosis can suffer a fracture with a small trauma that might not affect a woman with stronger bones. Fractures in the vertebral bones in the spine often don't require any trauma at all to occur. They may be first noticed when a woman has sudden back pain, or when an X ray is done for another reason. In clinical trial studies, women who are randomly assigned to take estrogen have less bone loss as they go through menopause and may be less likely to experience bone fractures, compared with women who are given placebo pills.

Estrogen and the Gallbladder

Estrogen also appears to be associated with the development of gallbladder stones. In a cohort study in California, Dr. Diane Pettiti and her colleagues found that women who currently took estrogen replacement therapy had a four times greater risk of having their gallbladder removed compared with women who had never taken estrogen. Almost all gallbladder removals are due to gallstones. Estrogen may cause gallstones to form by changing the composition of the bile that collects in the gall-bladder.

Progesterone

Other sex hormones are important in reproductive life and in breast development and growth. Progesterone, another hormone produced in the ovary, counteracts estrogens in some parts of the body, such as in the uterus, where it prevents the overstimulation of cells caused by estrogen. In the breast, however, progesterone seems to have a synergistic effect with estrogen. The highest rate of cells replicating themselves occurs at times of the month when a woman's progesterone levels are highest. Progesterone also causes the breast and other body tissue to retain water. Many women notice that their breasts are larger right before they get their periods—that is due to progesterone's effects. Women who have cysts (collections of fluid) in their breasts may notice that the cysts are larger before their periods. That is also due to the effects of progesterone. The effect of progesterone on risk for developing breast cancer is largely unknown. The Nurses' Health study, however, reported in 1995 that postmenopausal women who currently took a combination of proges-terone plus estrogen had a risk of breast cancer that was higher than that of women who took estrogen alone. Women who took estrogen and prog-esterone for the longest period of time had the greatest risk.

Testosterone and Other "Male" Hormones

Women produce androgens, or male hormones, in their ovaries and in their adrenal glands. These are released into the blood and circulate to all parts of the body. After menopause, the ovaries still produce andro-gens, but at a lower rate than before menopause. The adrenal glands con-tinue to produce androgens throughout life. So even in women who have had their ovaries removed, androgens are still produced. Androgens include hormones such as testosterone, DHEA (which stands for dehy-droepiandrosterone), and other male hormones and by-products of male hormone production and metabolism. Male hormones are important in the breast because they can be transformed into estrogen within the breast itself. There is a substance in the breast stromal tissue and fat called aromatase that converts testosterone and other male hormones into estrogen. Some women have more aromatase, or more active aromatase, than others. Women who have a lot of fat tissue in their breasts likely have more aromatase and therefore could make more estrogen out of the male hormones that reach the breast through the bloodstream. There have been several studies showing that women who have high levels of male hormones are at increased risk for developing breast cancer.

Other Hormones and the Breast

The cells and structures of the breast are under the control of other hormones such as thyroid hormone, growth hormones, insulin, and others. A few studies have looked at the levels of insulin in women who do and do not develop breast cancer. Early indications are that insulin may have a role in breast cancer, perhaps in promoting growth of breast tumors. Diabetic women who have high levels of insulin, however, are not necessarily at increased risk for breast cancer.

One intriguing hormone that may be related to breast cancer risk is called insulinlike growth hormone, or IGF. Despite its name, IGF is not an insulin; it is a growth hormone. This hormone is produced in many cells of the body and is involved in growth and development of many body structures. IGF circulates in the blood bound to a protein called insulinlike growth factor-binding protein, or IGFBP. Women who have high levels of IGFBP have lower levels of free or active IGF. IGF promotes the growth of tumor cells as well as normal cells. There are receptors for IGF in the breast, and IGF may be active in stimulating breast tissue during lactation. It is not surprising, then, that preliminary studies have found that women with high levels of IGF have an increased risk of developing breast cancer.

Many of these sex and other hormones are important in promoting the growth of breast cancers that have already occurred. Many breast cancers are estrogen-dependent; that is, the cancers grow under the influence of estrogen and regress when estrogen is withdrawn or blocked from acting. The drug tamoxifen works to treat some breast tumors by blocking the action of estrogen on the tumor cells. Before tamoxifen was available, doctors treated some women by removing their ovaries and adrenal glands, thereby blocking production of virtually all estrogen and male hormones.

Summary

- There are several different estrogens produced in women's bodies.
- Environment and biology affect how much and what kinds of estrogens are produced and how they are metabolized.
- Overweight and obese women make relatively high amounts of estrogen in their fat tissues through the activity of a substance called aromatase that is present in fat.
- Exercise reduces fat stores, so may reduce estrogen levels.
- Exercise increases production of proteins that bind estrogens, resulting in less estrogen activity.
- Estrogen affects many body parts and functions, as there are estrogen receptors in many body tissues.
- Estrogen has many beneficial effects on various body functions, including reproduction, pregnancy, and breast-feeding. It may benefit the heart, bones, and brain.
- Estrogen has several adverse effects, including increasing the risk for blood clots in the legs and lungs, gallbladder disease, cancer of the endometrium (uterine lining), and breast cancer.

9

Exercise as Part of the Treatment Plan for Breast Cancer Patients

Coping with a diagnosis of breast cancer can be an overwhelming process. Women undergoing treatment for breast cancer have to deal with significant physical and emotional side effects. Physical activity and exercise can play important roles in your healing and recovery process. In this chapter we discuss the many benefits of exercise for women going through treatment and after treatment. We begin with a description of exercises that can be done after surgery to improve arm and shoulder strength and mobility. We give some guidelines on preventing and dealing with lymphedema, a potential side effect of lymph node surgery for breast cancer. We suggest exercise as a way to fight the fatigue that commonly accompanies chemotherapy. Finally, we give some tips for gauging your capacity for exercise when you are feeling fatigued or ill during your treatment. We hope that this information will give you some assistance as you or your loved one is dealing with breast cancer treatment.

Exercise can be beneficial in the treatment of the physical effects of breast cancer and its treatment, through improved recovery from surgery, reduced fatigue, weight loss, and improved lymphatic flow. Exercise may also counter some of the emotional effects of breast cancer, such as poor body image, anxiety, loss of control, and depression.

Cancer patients commonly receive advice to rest and limit their activities during treatment. Such restriction of activities promotes muscular wasting and reduces functional capacity. You should begin physical rehabilitation programs as soon as pain and other complications of cancer therapy are controlled. Maintaining an exercise program throughout cancer treatment is not only safe but is also an effective way to manage symptoms and side effects.

Some breast cancer patients are accustomed to exercise while others have been relatively inactive either recently or all of their lives. Regardless of your exercise experience, you can benefit from the addition of physical activity to your breast cancer treatment plan. Patients who are used to vigorous activity often want to continue exercising during and after breast cancer treatment to maintain their lifestyle and feeling of well-being. Such exercise is generally safe, although it will likely need to be reduced for a time to avoid injuries and other problems. In contrast, patients who have been sedentary may need encouragement to begin a physical activity program at a time when fatigue and weakness from treatment make them want to take it easy. The appropriate type, intensity, and timing of exercise are different for each patient.

Women often do not know how to begin their recovery from cancer treatment. Many patients feel that they would benefit from an exercise program during or after treatment but are unsure about what would be best for them and how to start. Your basic exercise program might include walking, weight training, swimming, or yoga. Start off slowly and easily, gradually building stamina and strength. Ask your physician for recommendations or a referral to a physical therapy program at your clinic or hospital. A physical therapist can teach exercises to strengthen the arm and shoulder after surgery, as well as exercises to help regain the strength needed to perform your daily routine. In addition, physical therapists can provide information and instruction on lymphedema prevention and management. We describe sample exercise programs for breast cancer patients undergoing treatment later in the book. Be sure to talk with your physician if you are thinking of adopting any exercise program.

Benefits of Exercise in Breast Cancer Patients

Physical and Functional Health

- Improved healing and recovery from surgery
- Decreased lymphedema
- Higher energy levels, less fatigue

- Weight loss
- Decreased nausea
- Less pain

Psychological and Emotional Health

- Improved body and self-image
- Decreased anxiety
- Improved social interactions
- Better sense of control
- Improved depression and mood
- Better sleep patterns

Exercises After Surgery

Exercising after surgery will help you to regain motion and strength in your arm and shoulder. Physical activity is particularly important for breast cancer patients who have undergone axillary lymph node surgery. After a lymph node operation, you may experience limitations of arm and shoulder movements, and a loss of flexibility and strength in your arm and shoulder. It is important to work on gentle stretching of the shoulder and arm to gradually stretch the tissues back to their normal state.

Your exercises can begin slowly and gently shortly after surgery, and gradually you can become more active. If you have a surgical drain in place, your surgeon may advise you to wait until after this is removed to do any exercise. Your surgeon or physical therapist should monitor postoperative exercise for arm range of motion. While most patients regain their full range of motion in four to twelve weeks, some patients experience ongoing tightness and restricted motion.

You may do the exercises described below on the floor or on a bed. Do them at least once a day, and up to three times a day as you are recovering from surgery. In addition, use your arms as much as possible for activities such as reaching, combing your hair, eating, and washing and drying yourself. Try to let your arms swing from the shoulder when you walk. It may feel more comfortable to bend your elbows when walking briskly.

The following postsurgery exercises are provided by the University of Washington Breast Cancer Specialty Center.

Hand Clasp

- To start, you may want to put a pillow or two above your head for your arms to rest on.
- Lie on your back with your knees bent and your feet flat.
- Clasp your hands together and lift your arms overhead, elbows just slightly flexed.
- Stop when you feel tightness. Let the weight of your arms stretch your tissue a little more.
- Relax there for one minute. Each day, gradually increase the amount of time until you can do ten minutes with your arms all the way up.

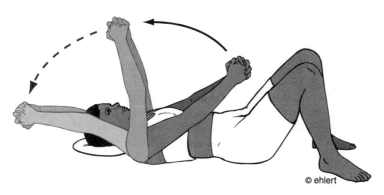

© ehlert

Figure 9.1. Hand clasp

Snow Angel

- To start, if you cannot get your elbow on the floor, put a pillow under your elbow.
- Lie on your back with your knees bent and feet flat.
- Move your arms out to the sides, keeping your elbows and wrists on the floor, preferably with your palms up.
- Move your arms up as high as you can, keeping your arms on the floor.

- Stay there one minute. Each day, gradually increase the amount of time until you can do ten minutes with your arms all the way up.

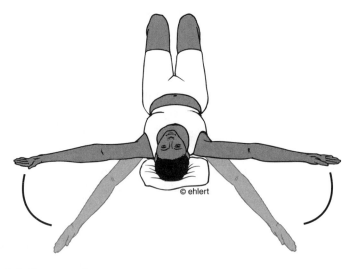

Figure 9.2. Snow angel

Daydream

- To start, you may want to put pillows under your elbows.
- Lie on your back with your knees bent and feet flat.
- Clasp your hands together behind your head.

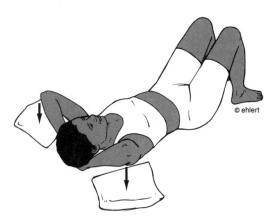

Figure 9.3. Daydream

- Let your elbows drop down to the floor or pillow.
- Keep them dropped for one minute to start. Each day, gradually increase the amount of time until you can do ten minutes with your elbows down.

Leaning on Your Hand

- Sit on the bed with your palm down at your side.
- Lean on your hand. Put more and more weight on it each day.
- Move your hand to different places farther away from you, out to the side, and behind you. Lean on your hand in these new positions, putting more weight on it.
- When this becomes easy for you, try crawling on your hands and knees.

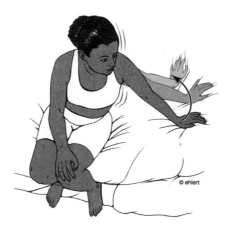

Figure 9.4. Leaning on your hand

Exercise as Therapy for Lymphedema

Lymphedema is an abnormal accumulation of lymphatic fluid (water and protein) in the soft tissue of the body. This is usually due to obstruction of lymphatic ducts. In breast cancer patients, lymphedema can cause swelling in the arm, hand, breast, or chest wall. Only a small percentage of breast cancer patients develop severe lymphedema, but many women experience mild symptoms, especially following significant arm activity. Regaining full motion and strength of the arm or shoulder blade follow-

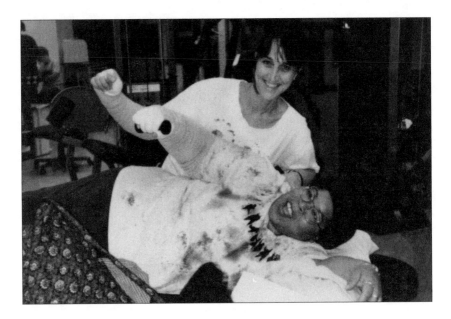

Physical therapist Marisa Perdomo (top) and De Nash (bottom) use exercise to manage their lymphedema. Photo: Lisa Talbott.

ing surgery through exercise is one of the best ways to decrease your risk of lymphedema.

Causes of Lymphedema

Factors that contribute to the onset of lymphedema include surgery or radiation therapy to the axillary lymph nodes. Surgery to the lymph node area under the arm causes decreased flow of lymphatic fluid as it passes through the remaining lymph nodes and ducts. Radiation to this area causes scarring in the lymph vessels, which also slows the flow of the lymphatic system in this region. Sometimes lymphedema is caused by breast cancer recurrence in the lymph nodes under the arm. (If you develop new swelling in your arm, it is important to see your oncologist as soon as possible, to make sure that you have not had a recurrence.)

Lymphedema may occur at any time following breast cancer treatment. There is no proven way to prevent lymphedema from occurring. Some women develop symptoms within the first year, and others first develop symptoms twenty years later. Infections in the hand or arm on the side of the breast surgery may trigger the onset of lymphedema. Aircraft flight has been linked to the onset of lymphedema in some breast cancer patients, likely due to decreased cabin pressure. The risk of developing lymphedema after breast surgery or radiation varies widely, depending on the type of treatment and the patient's body size and shape. Being overweight increases the likelihood of developing arm swelling due to differences in lymph volume and flow.

Symptoms of Lymphedema

The most common symptom of lymphedema is arm swelling—fluid accumulates to the point that the skin is actually stretched. Other symptoms can include heaviness, weakness, tingling, numbness, achiness, loss of motor coordination, or pain in the affected arm. Initially, the swelling or other symptoms might fluctuate with activity. Many people believe that since the swelling goes away with rest, they don't need treatment. However, this is exactly when treatment should be started. If caught in the very early stages, treatment is less time-consuming, and results are obtained much more quickly.

Reducing Your Risk for Lymphedema

Some doctors recommend seeing a physical therapist before or immediately after surgery to learn ways to reduce your chances of developing lymphedema and other postsurgery problems. Regaining full motion and strength of the arm or shoulder blade following surgery, along with the early treatment of infections, is the best way to decrease your risk of lymphedema. You should learn how to prevent injuries and infections and what to do should one occur.

Here are some ways to decrease your risk of developing lymphedema after breast cancer surgery:

- Avoid trauma to the affected side (bruising, cuts, sunburn or other burns, sports injuries, insect bites, cat scratches).
- Treat infections of the affected arm early. Your doctor will prescribe appropriate antibiotics. (Some women carry a prescrip-

tion with them when they travel, in case infection develops on the road.)

- Use an electric razor rather than a safety razor to avoid nicks.
- Try to avoid injections or blood drawing in the affected arm. (It may be necessary to have blood drawn in this arm during chemotherapy, so that the chemotherapy itself can be given in the unaffected arm).
- Have blood pressure checks in the unaffected arm.
- Avoid lifting heavy objects that would cause you strain. (Weight lifting for exercise is safe for most women but must be individualized. See Chapter 18 for more information.)
- Avoid vigorous, repetitive movements against resistance.
- Do not wear tight jewelry or elastic bands around affected fingers or arms.
- Avoid cutting cuticles when manicuring hands.
- Keep your weight down.
- Consider wearing a compression garment on your arm when you fly.
- Avoid tobacco, alcohol, and salt.

Treating Lymphedema

Specially trained physical therapists, occupational therapists, and massage therapists treat lymphedema. Many insurance plans cover lymphedema treatment services as long as a licensed therapist provides the treatment. A lymphedema treatment plan usually includes some combination of exercise, massage, and bandaging or compression garments.

These are some ways that lymphedema can be treated:

- Manual lymphatic drainage (massage)
- Bandaging and compression garments (sleeves, stockings)
- Exercises
- Proper skin and nail care

Manual lymphatic drainage involves gentle massage, starting with the chest and moving to the arm. This should be done once or twice a day. A therapist can teach you or a family member how to perform this massage. The goal is to open obstructed lymph vessels so that the fluid from the swollen arm has someplace to go. Bandages are wrapped around the arm immediately after each massage to prevent the lymph that has been drained out from reaccumulating. The bandages are worn overnight until the next treatment session. Compression garments include gloves and sleeves that have been custom-made to fit each patient. They can be worn daily or during activities known to increase arm swelling, such as during physical activity, gardening, and flying. Exercises are done with the bandages or compression garments in place. This forces the muscles to contract against the nonyielding wraps and results in an outflow of lymph from the arm. Skin and nail care help keep the arm clean and free of infection. A good skin lotion should be applied once or twice daily to prevent cuts due to dryness and chafing.

Exercise to Decrease Treatment Side Effects

Research suggests that maintaining physical activity during breast cancer treatment can decrease pain, nausea, weight gain, and fatigue, while increasing energy. Maintaining your strength during treatment with exercise and physical activity improves your ability to perform activities of daily living, including personal hygiene, household chores, leisure activities, and occupational requirements.

Fatigue and Energy Levels

Many breast cancer patients feel that fatigue is the most distressing side effect of treatment. Cancer-related fatigue affects 40–90 percent of patients undergoing treatment for cancer. Energy levels during treatment are different for every breast cancer patient, depending on the extent of the disease and the treatment received. Fatigue may persist in breast cancer survivors years after treatment ends and can result in significant decreases in quality of life. Continued low energy levels have been reported as long as twenty months after radiation therapy for breast cancer.

What Causes Fatigue?

There are many reasons for fatigue in patients undergoing treatment for breast cancer. Low red blood cell counts due to chemotherapy or radiation therapy result in anemia, a major cause of fatigue. Other reasons for fatigue, including anxiety, depression, poor nutrition, and disrupted sleep patterns. In addition, the drugs and radiation therapy can cause fatigue. Finally, feelings of fatigue can be the result of emotional stress, not enough support from others, or depression or anxiety.

Causes of Fatigue in Cancer Patients

- Side effects of treatment, medications, procedures
- Inadequate nutrition
- Infection/fever
- Pain
- Anemia
- Stress, depression, anxiety
- Sleep disturbances
- Excessive inactivity, rest, or immobility
- Cancer progression

Evaluating and Managing Fatigue

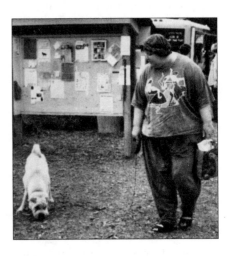

A natural response to feeling fatigued is to decrease physical activity. When patients complain of being fatigued, health care providers often recommend additional rest and decreased activity. Over time, this leads to decreased functional capacity and less ability to tolerate exercise and even normal activity. It is discouraging not to have your usual energy and sometimes not

During her cancer treatment, Marcia Vickery used short walks with her dog, Comedy, to manage her fatigue. Photo: Julie Gralow.

to be able to do even basic tasks. Often you will have to manage your fatigue by making some adjustments in your routine. Prioritize your tasks and make sure you are doing the most important ones when you still have energy. You don't have to give up important activities; just reduce some of them and save your energy for those things you consider priorities. If possible, extra help with shopping, cooking, and child care can be a big help. Many women find that taking very short naps during the day improves quality of sleep at night and also helps raise energy levels.

How to Assess Your Fatigue

- How frequently do you feel fatigued?
- How severe is your fatigue (on a scale of 0–10)?
- At what time of day is your fatigue the most intense?
- Do you feel fatigued after receiving medical treatment? If yes, when?
- Keep an activities journal; use the journal to develop strategies for managing your fatigue.
- What activities make you tired?
- What prevents or relieves your tiredness?
- What activities must you do?
- What activities do you like to do?
- What activities could you delegate to others?

Maintain some exercise program if at all possible. When women don't feel well they often stop exercising altogether. Research is showing, however, that maintaining some level of mild exercise (walking, swimming, and yoga) may actually increase energy levels in women undergoing cancer treatments. Investigators have looked at exercise as a strategy for treating fatigue. In one study, breast cancer patients undergoing radiation therapy were randomized to six weeks of exercise versus usual care. Symptoms of fatigue, anxiety, and sleep disturbances were significantly lower in the women participating in the exercise group. Another study evaluated the impact of exercise on fatigue by keeping track of how much physical activity and exercise breast cancer patients got each week while undergoing treatment. The more minutes of exercise per week predicted less fatigue.

If you are significantly fatigued or otherwise affected by anemia, there are ways to increase the red cell blood counts. Red blood cell transfusions can increase your hematocrit. Erythropoetin (Epogen, Procrit) is a growth stimulator for red blood cells given by injection that can help boost the hematocrit and decrease anemia. If you are experiencing fatigue, make sure to tell your physician. Fatigue can often be treated successfully.

How to Help Manage Fatigue

- Try to sleep longer at night.
- Schedule naps during the day whenever possible.
- Set your priorities—don't try to do everything you did before you began breast cancer treatment.
- Ask for assistance when you need it. Accept help from friends and family when it is offered.
- Try to eat a balanced diet.
- Include regular physical activity.

✍ Exercise Benefits Pain, Nausea, and Other Treatment Side Effects

Several studies have found that physical activity during and after breast cancer treatment can reduce symptoms of nausea, pain, diarrhea, insomnia, and weight gain. One study evaluated the possible benefits of a walking program during radiation therapy for breast cancer. Women maintained an individualized, self-paced, home-based walking program through their radiation treatment. A control group received usual care. The exercise group did significantly better in both physical functioning and symptom intensity. Some studies have shown that exercise can improve blood cell counts and natural immunity, which could theoretically lead to decreased infections during chemotherapy, although this latter has not been proved in scientific studies.

The effect of exercise on chemotherapy-induced nausea has been investigated in one study in which forty-five women who were receiving chemotherapy for stage II breast cancer were asked to perform moderate aerobic activity using exercycles. Compared to a control group of women who did not exercise, nausea was significantly less in the exercise group.

Cancer-related pain can be reduced through a regular program of physical activity, as shown in several studies. This may be due to better overall conditioning and muscle strength, or decreased stress and emotional factors. Exercise is known to increase the release of endorphins, the body's natural painkillers.

Weight gain occurs in more than 70 percent of women undergoing treatment for breast cancer. Although you might think chemotherapy should cause weight loss due to nausea and decreased appetite, this is not generally the case. Exercise can help guard against excessive weight gain from the time you are diagnosed. Controlling weight gain can have emotional and psychological benefits. It may also improve your chances for long-term survival, since women who gain weight after diagnosis have poorer survival compared to women whose weight remains stable.

Psychological and Emotional Benefits of Exercise

Regular physical activity improves mood, body image, self-concept, and sleep patterns. Exercise can decrease anxiety, tension, anger, pessimism, depression, and feelings of helplessness in cancer patients. Studies investigating the relationship between exercise and well-being in women with breast cancer have demonstrated that women who exercise have a significantly higher quality of life. When women feel they have control of their bodies again they are empowered to get back to work or school and take on physical or emotional challenges, including strengthening personal relationships. Physical exercise may also have an impact on the spirituality dimension of well-being. Women who exercise are also more likely to do breast self-exams and take care of their health problems as they arise.

It doesn't require a significant time commitment to achieve emotional and psychological benefit from exercise. A study looked at the effect of aerobic exercise on self-esteem, depression, and anxiety symptoms among breast cancer survivors. Women with breast cancer were asked to exercise for thirty to forty minutes, four times per week. Significantly decreased depression and anxiety were seen after just ten weeks. This research showed that the improved psychological state resulting from exercise gives patients hope and improves the ability to cope with and adapt to stress. In addition, women in exercise studies have reported higher levels of satisfaction with their bodies. However, you don't need to do this amount of exercise to experience benefits. Any physical activity, such as one group class a week (yoga, for example) or a walk with a friend a couple of times per week, can improve your mood and increase your energy.

Guidelines for Safe Exercise While Undergoing Cancer Treatment

It is generally safe to exercise during your cancer treatment and recovery. In fact, exercise can be an effective way to manage some of the side effects of treatment. If you were physically active before your breast cancer diagnosis, you will have different goals and abilities from women who were relatively inactive. Exercise programs should be modified to reflect your functional ability and activity tolerance. Be sure to discuss your

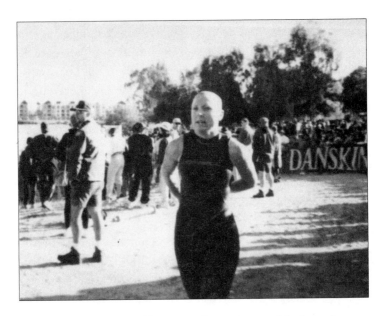

Athlete Kristin Bauersfeld continued to exercise safely throughout her cancer treatment by maintaining lower heart rates during training and races. Photo: Lisa Talbott.

exercise plans with your physician before starting an exercise program and throughout your cancer treatment.

Find out how much exercise and activity you can tolerate by starting with small goals. Exercise for short amounts of time (five to ten minutes) a few times each day, with rest periods in between. By gradually reducing the rest periods and increasing the exercise periods, you can work up to thirty minutes of continuous exercise.

Set goals and stick with them. Keep an exercise diary. Consider consulting a trainer or physical therapist to help set realistic goals and to monitor progress.

Exercise Intensity

Start slowly to avoid injuries to muscles, tendons, joints, and bones. Gradually increase the intensity and duration of the exercise. Monitoring your heart rate by checking your pulse or with a heart rate monitor is a good way to tell if you're staying at appropriate exercise intensity levels. During treatment, it is best to stay below 65 percent of your maximum heart rate (see Chapter 14) to reduce fatigue symptoms. (Some research suggests that when cancer patients exercise above 65 percent of their maximum heart rate, fatigue levels may increase.) After treatment, above 65 percent is encouraged (60–80 percent). Exercising above 80 percent of your maximum heart rate is not recommended for three to six months following treatment. If you were in good athletic condition before treatment, higher heart rates may be acceptable sooner.

Blood Counts

Patients undergoing chemotherapy often have temporary depressions in their blood cell counts. Normal counts for these cells are given in Table 9-1. Your blood counts should serve as a guide to your exercise plans while on treatment. If your platelet count is below 50,000, gentle exercise and stretching is okay, but more intense exercise could cause bruising or bleeding. For a hemoglobin count of less than 10, most exercise is okay, but fatigue will set in quickly due to the body's decreased ability to deliver oxygen throughout the body, including the muscles. If your absolute neutrophil count is less than 1,000, exercise at home and avoid group exercise: your immune system is temporarily compromised. Don't use community exercise equipment (including swimming pools), and don't exercise in an environment that may expose you to infection.

Table 9.1. Normal Blood Counts

BLOOD ELEMENT	NORMAL COUNT (will vary slightly from lab to lab)
Platelets (important for blood clotting)	150,000–400,000 µL (micro liter)
Hemoglobin (a measure of red blood cell health—low value equals anemia)	11.5–15.5 g/dL (grams per deeiliter)
Neutrophils (white blood cells important for fighting infection)	1.8–7.0 thousand µL (micro liter)

Remember, inadequate diet or insufficient fluid intake may cause adverse symptoms and compromise exercise capabilities during and after treatment.

When You Should Not Exercise

Exercise during treatment is not recommended if you are experiencing any of the following symptoms:

- Irregular pulse or resting pulse higher than 100 beats per minute
- Recurring leg pain or cramps
- Chest pain
- Acute onset of nausea during exercise
- Disorientation/confusion
- Dizziness, blurred vision, fainting
- Bone, back, or neck pain of recent onset
- Extreme paleness or anemia
- Illness with fever

- Sudden onset of shortness of breath, muscular weakness, or unusual fatigue

It is important to pay close attention to your body's signals. These may see like obvious symptoms that would keep you from exercising. However, during cancer treatment, it is sometimes difficult to know what is normal and what could be a problem. Don't be afraid to ask your doctor or nurse about exercising. He or she will likely be pleased to know that you are feeling well enough to exercise!

Summary

- Exercise can be an important part of your treatment plan.
- Exercise can reduce fatigue, speed recovery from surgery, prevent weight gain from chemotherapy, decrease risk for lymphedema, and counter some negative emotional effects of breast cancer diagnosis and treatment.
- Take care not to exceed your body's current capabilities to exercise. Don't push yourself too hard. Start gradually and be aware of your body's signals that it is getting fatigued from the exercise.
- Performing special exercises can prevent and treat lymphedema, the generalized arm swelling that can occur as a result of breast cancer therapy.
- Fatigue can be managed with exercise and other techniques.

10

Exercise to Reduce Risk of
Breast Cancer Recurrence

In this chapter we are charting new territory. There has been very little research on the health effects of exercise in breast cancer patients. Therefore, much of what we say is based on extrapolation of data from individuals without breast cancer and from our knowledge of the biology of breast cancer. In this chapter, we present information on the association between being overweight or obese and poor risk for survival among breast cancer patients. We describe what little research has been done on exercise and breast cancer prognosis. We talk about the potential role of diet in recovery from breast cancer and the various studies now going on to answer open questions on nutrition and breast cancer prognosis. We talk about how body fat and exercise might affect breast cancer prognosis. We describe the available research on exercise and quality of life. Finally, we give recommendations on how you can use exercise and nutrition to control weight and improve your well-being after a diagnosis of breast cancer.

When you first were diagnosed with breast cancer, your doctor may have given you some idea of your likely prognosis given your age, type of cancer, and whether it had already spread when you were diagnosed. These prognosis statistics usually take into account the tumor characteristics, your age, and whether you have passed through menopause. The tumor characteristics that affect prognosis include size of tumor, number of lymph nodes that have cancer cells in them, whether the cancer has spread to other parts of the body, and whether hormone receptors are present. Scientists and doctors now have learned more about specific tumor cell characteristics that can predict prognosis and are starting to pass that information on to the patient as well as designing treatment plans according to tumor characteristics. HER2neu is an example of a newly discovered tumor characteristic that doctors use to decide on treatment and to make predictions about prognosis. However, very few doctors are currently using information about patient body weight to predict prognosis, and most are not using weight information to decide which therapies to use (other than to select drug dosages).

Overweight, Obesity, and Breast Cancer Survival

For the past two decades, breast cancer scientists have been finding that women who are obese or overweight at diagnosis have a poorer prognosis from their breast cancer compared with thinner women. Almost two dozen studies have followed breast cancer patients after diagnosis and have found that women who are the heaviest—have the highest body mass—have a two to three times greater risk of dying of their breast cancer after five or ten years of follow-up. A British study published in 1998 followed 2,455 stage I and II breast cancer patients who were under age seventy at diagnosis. They found that women who weighed 132 pounds or more at diagnosis were 70 percent more likely to die from breast cancer within five years after diagnosis compared with women who weighed less than 132 pounds. In contrast, the risk of their dying of causes other than breast cancer did not differ by weight. A 1997 publication of Canadian researchers detailed their study in which they followed 1,169 stage I, II and III breast cancer patients. They found those women with body mass index of 22.8 or greater had more than two times the risk of dying within ten years compared with lighter women. The effect of body mass, however, was limited to women who did not have cancer in their lymph nodes at diagnosis. Australian scientists reported in 1996 on a study of 1,138 breast cancer patients who had negative lymph nodes; they found a 10 percent better prognosis in patients whose body mass index was under 28 compared with heavier women. Norwegian scientists reported in 1996 that their study of 1,238 breast cancer patients also found a poorer survival with increased weight.

Obese patients were 40 percent more likely to die from breast cancer within an average of about five years compared with thin women, although this was true only of women with certain types of tumors (those whose tumors were responsive to estrogen). Several additional studies of this sort have been done in other countries. Most agree with these findings: Overweight and obese women have poorer survival rates than thin women do.

At first, researchers thought that women who were heavier were not getting diagnosed as early as lighter women were. It is true that overweight and obese women tend to have more advanced disease when they are first diagnosed with breast cancer. Their tumors are larger, are more aggressive, and have more often spread to the lymph nodes, compared with the tumors of thinner women. However, many of the studies were able to control for these factors related to type of breast cancer. Even after accounting for these differences in tumor characteristics, women who are overweight or obese continue to have poorer survival rates compared with lighter women. So what could be the reasons for this, and what does it mean for you if you have breast cancer?

Studies of Exercise and Breast Cancer Survival

There has been only one small study looking at the effect of exercise on survival from breast cancer. This study included only 451 patients, and it did not find an effect of activity on survival. A major flaw of this study, however, was that it looked only at the activities a woman was doing before her diagnosis of breast cancer. Most women change their physical activity habits during breast cancer treatment and afterward. We do not know from this study whether a woman who starts exercising after a diagnosis of breast cancer and becomes fitter has an improved chance of long-term survival. The study was also too small to say definitively whether exercise affects survival. A third serious problem with the study was that the patients were followed for only an average of four years after diagnosis. Several thousand patients would need to be followed for more than five years to determine survival effects.

Fortunately, there are some studies underway to look at various lifestyle and other factors that might affect survival. One study that we

are doing at the Fred Hutchinson Cancer Research Center
is called the Health, Eating,
Activity, and Lifestyle (HEAL)
study. It is being conducted in
western Washington, Southern
California, and New Mexico.
We are enrolling approximately
1,200 women within four to
twelve months after diagnosis
of breast cancer, collecting
information and making measurements, and following them
forward over time to determine
the effect of exercise, diet,
weight patterns, body fat distribution, and blood hormones on
breast cancer recurrence and
survival. One unique aspect of

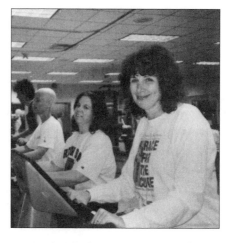

*Erica Shrack (front) and Christine
Halfon (behind) participate in Team
Survivor's group conditioning class at
the Exercise Training Center at the
University of Washington Roosevelt
Clinic. Photo: Lisa Talbott.*

the study is that there are large numbers of minority women involved,
particularly African-American and Mexican-American women. The first
results of this study will be available in 2004 or so. Other studies are
underway in other centers in the United States and in Canada to look at
the effect of exercise on breast cancer survival.

Diet and Survival from Breast Cancer

Few studies have looked at the association between specific dietary
habits and breast cancer prognosis. A recently published study interviewed, measured, and followed 472 women who were treated for early-
stage breast cancer in New York. The researchers found that patients
who ate the most meat, butter, and margarine, and drank the most
beer had almost two times greater risk of having a recurrence of their
cancer compared with women who seldom ate these foods. Similarly,
a high intake of these foods and drink increased risk of dying from
breast cancer.

How Exercise and Weight Control Can Reduce Breast Cancer Recurrence and Improve Survival

Most breast cancers are estrogen-dependent, which means that estrogen stimulates the growth and spread of the breast cancer cells. Furthermore, removing sources of estrogen is an effective treatment for these cancers. Removing estrogen can be in the form of surgical removal of the ovaries and the adrenal glands. Estrogen can also be "removed" by use of a drug that interferes with its action. Tamoxifen is one drug that works by keeping estrogen away from the breast cancer cells. Since estrogen is so potent at promoting the growth and spread of many breast cancer cells, and since its removal through surgery is an effective treatment, it makes sense that lowering estrogen through exercise, diet, and reduction of body fat could also be a useful therapy. As we described in Chapter 6, exercise can lower estrogen levels in teens and young women by affecting the pituitary gland and causing changes to menstrual patterns. Exercise may lower estrogen levels in postmenopausal women by reducing body fat, which is the major site of estrogen production in older women.

Moderate levels of daily physical activity can improve the immune system. Although we do not know much about how the immune system fights the spread of cancer, we do know that people whose immune systems are deficient have high risk for aggressive cancers. For example, persons with HIV have a high risk for cancers of the lymph system and the cervix. There is much work going on to find vaccines that can stimulate a woman's immune system to better fight her cancer cells. In the laboratory, certain white blood cells, called natural killer cells, when activated can stop growth of breast cancer cells. Other cells called macrophages may help to fight cancer cells. Both of these types of cells secrete substances that also may fight breast cancer cells. So we believe that a strong immune system is likely involved in increasing a breast cancer patient's chance for long-term survival.

Other Benefits of Exercise That Can Improve Breast Cancer Survival and Quality of Life

Breast cancer patients who are actively involved in their treatment and who seek and use social support have better survival than do women who

Exercise to Reduce Risk of Breast Cancer Recurrence   127

are not so involved. Several different interventions to improve quality of life have been tested, and most appear to improve patients' subjective experiences and feelings. Relaxation training, meditation, education, social support groups, counseling or psychotherapy, and music therapy have all been found to increase breast cancer patients' quality of life, at least to a degree. The effects of these interventions have been small, however, indicating that more is needed to help patients through their experiences. In addition, these interventions have little effect if any on patients' ability to function physically. Recent research indicates that the ability to function in activities of daily living is the most important aspect of quality of life for many breast cancer patients.

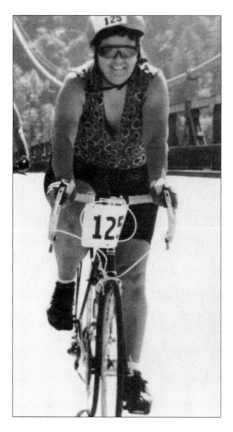

Turning forty and going through breast cancer treatment motivated Teresa Martinez to start biking. She averages fifty miles a week and completed a number of 100- and 200-mile bike tours.

About a half dozen experimental studies have assessed the effect of an exercise intervention on quality of life in breast cancer patients. Most of the studies have been very small, and most have been of short duration (ten to twelve weeks or less). Four studies measured exercise effect on physical functioning, and all showed a benefit. One study of forty-five stage II breast cancer patients found that supervised stationary bicycling three times weekly for ten weeks increased functional capacity while a control group of patients had no change in functional capacity. Other studies found that regular exercise increased the distance a woman could walk in six minutes, which indicates gains in cardiovascular fitness and muscle function. A study of forty-six stage I and II breast cancer patients found that women who were assigned to a walking program (twenty to thirty minutes, four to five times per week for six weeks) had decreased fatigue, anxiety, and sleep problems compared with control women who did not walk. A small study of fourteen stage I and II patients found that exercise improved psychological adjustment and reduced symptoms, compared with controls. Definitive results await larger and better studies, but these studies point to a potential role for exercise in improving quality of life, functional ability, and, perhaps, prognosis.

Other Health Benefits That Are Important to Breast Cancer Patients and Survivors

As we explain in Chapter 12, breast cancer patients who are menopausal or become menopausal from treatment can have magnified menopausal symptoms and effects. The symptoms may decrease over time, and the abrupt early menopause may actually protect against further breast cancer by reducing estrogen levels. The reduced estrogen levels, however, can increase a woman's risk for other diseases such as heart disease and osteoporosis. For this reason, and because most breast cancer patients live for many years after a diagnosis, you should continue to monitor your overall health. Exercise is an excellent way to promote cardiovascular, bone, and mental health.

How to Reduce Excess Body Fat and Avoid Fat Gain After Diagnosis

As we have discussed throughout this book, exercise is the best method for reducing body fat and keeping it off. Restricting calories may be necessary in addition if you are very overweight or if you are not exercising at a high level. We do not recommend that you try to restrict calories while you are undergoing therapy, however, since this could cause deficiency of critical nutrients. We also do not advise you to use calorie restriction alone to reduce excess body fat. Restricting calories alone will cause you to lose weight, but you will lose muscle in addition to fat, which will leave you feeling weak and more fatigued than you were before you dieted.

There are some dietary changes you can make that will help you lose excess fat, maintain muscle, and increase your energy levels after a diagnosis of breast cancer. These changes can be done during and after treatment. They simply involve making choices based on what will nourish your body. We recommend that you increase your intake of vegetable and fruits to a minimum of eight servings per day. One serving equals one half cup of cooked vegetables or one piece of fruit or one 6-ounce glass of juice. By increasing your intake of vegetables and fruits, you will be doing several things:

- Increasing your intake of vitamins and some minerals
- Increasing fiber
- Filling up with lower-calorie foods, helping you to feel full and satisfied
- Increasing water intake since vegetables and fruits hold water

Another recommendation is to limit your intake of sweets and high-fat foods. Don't eliminate them—just don't make them the mainstay of your diet.

Finally, we recommend that you know your body and what it needs at the moment, and eat to supply those needs. If you concentrate on eating for food's nutrition, you will be more likely to feel full from the nutritious foods you are choosing and less likely to fill up on junk food. For example, if your white blood cell count is low, then make sure that you are eating foods that help to improve your immune system (folate, vitamin B^{12}, zinc, and iron). This may not make your white count rise faster, but it may help other parts of your immune system function better while your count recovers. If you are anemic, make sure that you have adequate iron intake. The anemia from chemotherapy is not from iron deficiency. However, if you add iron deficiency on top of anemia from chemotherapy, the result is even more fatigue. Talk with a nutritionist if you want to learn more about what good nutrition can do for you as you are recovering from breast cancer.

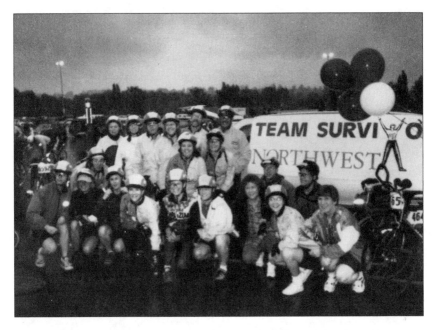

Team Survivor Northwest members, volunteers, friends, and family at the start of the 1998 Seattle to Portland Bike Classic

Increasing Your Exercise After Diagnosis

If you want to increase your exercise after diagnosis for any reason, check with your doctor first regarding any concerns he or she has for your own situation. Read Chapter 9 and Chapters 14 through 21 to learn techniques for exercise. Look for the special tips for breast cancer patients and survivors throughout these chapters. Finally, read Chapter 13 to learn how other breast cancer survivors have used exercise to improve their lives after their diagnosis.

Summary

- Women with breast cancer who are overweight or obese have poorer short- and long-term survival rates compared with thinner women.

- Part of the effect of overweight and obesity on survival may be related to diet.
- Exercise (and diet) have a potential to reduce breast cancer recurrence because both can lower blood estrogen levels, which have been shown to increase breast cancer risk at high levels.
- Exercise has been shown to improve various aspects of quality of life and physical functioning in breast cancer patients.
- Most women survive their breast cancer and can therefore expect to live about as long as women without breast cancer. For this reason, breast cancer patients should take care of their overall health. Exercise can be an important part of that care.
- Exercise can be helpful for overweight or obese women wanting to reduce extra fat mass after they complete their breast cancer therapy.
- Check with your doctor before you start or increase an exercise program if you are a breast cancer patient in current or recently completed treatment.

11

Other Ways to Decrease Recurrence of Breast Cancer

Once you have completed the primary phase of your treatment, a regimen of follow-up care will begin and will continue for your lifetime. The purpose is to monitor the healing process and watch for a possible recurrence of cancer. Even after treatment ends, you may continue to fear that you will have a recurrence. You can get some reassurance that the possibility of breast cancer recurrence becomes less likely with the passage of time. In this chapter, we describe several things you can do to help your long-term prognosis after a diagnosis of breast cancer, including getting optimal treatment, getting good follow-up so that any recurrences are caught early, and getting regular breast screening. We recommend some other things that might help your prognosis, although the scientific research to support them is lacking. These include diet, minimizing alcohol use, and controlling excess body fat. We describe some new research that is being done on diet and antiestrogen medications (called SERMs) on breast cancer recurrence and survival.

Many women find that their follow-up appointments are times when their fear of recurrence and anxiety surface. Even the approach of the five- and ten-year milestones might make you feel more anxious than secure. Taking control of your health and working with your health care team will result in your optimal physical and emotional well-being. Adopting a health maintenance program and healthy lifestyle can reduce your risk of breast cancer recurrence and improve your overall health.

The following suggestions are based on breast cancer specialists' observations on what improves survival in their patients.

1. *Your breast cancer treatment.* Your first line of defense after a diagnosis of breast cancer is getting the best and most complete treatment that is appropriate for your type of cancer. Good primary treatment of the breast cancer with surgery, radiation, and systemic therapy is the best way to decrease the likelihood of recurrence. Many doctors and scientists believe that any patient with invasive breast cancer can have some cancer cells in her blood or lymph that are too few in number to show up in standard tests. The best chance of eradicating all cancer cells is at a time when they are microscopic and undetectable.

2. *Your follow-up after diagnosis.* Get regular checkups after the completion of your breast cancer treatment. Have your doctor outline a follow-up program, including the frequency of physical examinations, mammograms, blood work, and X rays. Your follow-up program will depend on your stage at diagnosis, the treatment you received, and the presence or absence of lingering treatment side effects.

3. *Find new cancers and recurrences early.* Consider new breast cancer imaging and detection techniques. If your breasts are difficult to follow by mammogram and physical exam due to denseness, scarring, or other factors, you may be a candidate for breast ultrasound, magnetic resonance imaging (MRI), or nuclear medicine studies and techniques. Serum tumor markers such as CA2.29 (CA 15-3), CEA, and CA-125 are used in following some patients for recurrence. These tests detect proteins circulating in the blood that can be shed from tumor cells as well as some normal cells in the body. Tumor marker tests can be insensitive and nonspecific, and have not been shown to improve survival from breast cancer.

4. *Adopt a healthy lifestyle.* We have discussed at length the importance of exercise and maintaining an appropriate body weight, avoiding obesity, and eating a healthy diet. These

basic health maintenance measures will help you feel better, lower your risk of a wide variety of other health problems, and may decrease your risk of breast cancer recurrence.

5. *Understand your risk.* If your family history suggests an inherited predisposition to breast cancer, talk to a genetic counselor and become informed. You may be at high risk for a second breast cancer, ovarian cancer, or other cancers. Understanding your genetic risk for cancer can help you make decisions about prophylactic surgeries and other cancer risk reduction measures. Genetic testing can now be done for BRCA1 and BRCA2, and other genes associated with breast cancer risk will undoubtedly be found in the future. All breast cancer survivors, regardless of their genetic risk, have a higher than average risk of developing a second breast cancer, in addition to their risk of recurrence of the original breast cancer. For this reason it is imperative that you get regular mammograms and clinical breast exams at the intervals that your oncologist or breast surgeon prescribes.

6. *Minimize environmental risk factors.* There is little definitive data about which environmental factors may contribute to breast cancer risk, but it is generally a good idea to avoid excessive exposure to radiation and pesticides.

7. *Consider participating in clinical trials.* Significant advances in breast cancer treatment and survival have been the result of carefully designed clinical trials. There are always new drugs and other treatment strategies in all stages of clinical testing. Some studies have shown that patients who are treated in clinical trials have better survival compared with women who do not enroll in clinical trials. Ask your doctor, nurse, or local hospital or cancer center if you are a candidate for a trial related to treatment or survivorship issues.

8. *Take care of your emotional health.* A study of stage IV breast cancer patients at Stanford University found significantly improved survival in patients who participated in support groups compared to a control group of patients who received usual care. Other studies have shown that women who participate in support groups learn skills and

develop social supports that assist them in adapting to breast cancer.

Breast Exams, Mammograms, and Other Imaging in Breast Cancer Survivors

Since your risk of developing a new breast cancer, or a recurrent cancer, is higher than for women who have not had breast cancer, it is particularly important for you to get regular breast screening. The screening methods are similar to what you had when you were diagnosed with cancer, but your doctor may want to do some additional tests depending on your type of breast cancer and what your breasts look like on mammograms.

Breast Self-Exam

Breast self-exam begins with the pads of your fingers (with the first three fingers held flat), not the nails. Palpate all the breast tissue from the collarbone (clavicle) to the breastbone (sternum) and extending into the underarm area. If you have had a mastectomy, palpate along the scar for any changes. A good breast exam includes examining breasts in front of a mirror as well as while lying down. Many women examine their breasts in the shower—wet skin may allow you to pick up smaller lumps or changes. The more you examine your breasts over time, the more familiar you will become with their contours. Any change should be followed up with your health care provider.

Clinical Breast Exam

A thorough exam by your health care provider is recommended every three to six months for the first five years after your diagnosis of breast cancer, then annually after that. However, your doctor may recommend a different schedule for you.

Mammograms

Regular mammogram screening can reduce your risk of dying from breast cancer. You should make sure to get screened at whatever interval your doctor recommends. If you had a lumpectomy, mammograms of the affected breast every six months are recommended for one to two years after diagnosis. Mammograms of the unaffected breast should be done every year. Bring your prior mammograms (if they were done at another facility) and be prepared with your breast health history; this will help with fast and accurate interpretation of your mammogram results.

Nutrition

A growing body of research supports the effect of diet on health. Obesity, high-fat diets, and high alcohol intake have all been implicated in increasing the risk of developing breast cancer. There may also be a link between these dietary factors, particularly being overweight, and a higher risk of breast cancer recurrence. Excess fat stores can raise the levels of estrogens in the blood that can promote the growth of breast cancer cells. Some researchers have suggested that monounsaturated fats, which are present in high amounts in olive oil and canola oil, may not increase risk for breast cancer.

There is evidence that breast cancer is less common in countries where the typical diet is high in soy. Isoflavones, which are sometimes called phytoestrogens or plant estrogens, are found in soy foods. They have properties similar to human estrogen but are much weaker. Isoflavones may have beneficial health effects, including decreasing symptoms associated with menopause such as hot flashes and decreasing heart disease and osteoporosis. Studies looking at dietary intake of soy and the risk of breast cancer suggest that isoflavones may have a protective effect against breast cancer. Laboratory studies have shown conflicting data, with breast cancer stimulation or inhibition depending on which cell lines, type of isoflavone, and dose of these agents are used. Phytoestrogens can be very helpful in managing menopausal symptoms in breast cancer survivors.

However, some doctors feel that women with estrogen-receptor positive breast cancer or those who are on tamoxifen should minimize their intake of isoflavones until we have a better understanding of the effect of phytoestrogens on breast tumors.

Dr. Julie Gralow and her colleagues at the University of Washington and the Fred Hutchinson Cancer Research Center are looking at the effect of a soy supplement on breast proliferation, menopausal symptoms, and other outcomes in postmenopausal women with breast cancer. This is a small pilot study, but it should give some important information that can help in the design of larger future studies.

Some researchers have focused on fruits and vegetables and their contents of vitamins and minerals as links between diet and breast cancer risk. Vitamins contain substances called antioxidants, which work to repair the cell's DNA after it has been damaged by a number of causes, including X rays, sunlight, and chemicals. Some vitamins, such as the vitamin A–related retinoids and beta-carotene, can regulate the growth of cancer cells. There are clinical trials underway testing the effects of some of these vitamins in breast cancer patients.

One recently published Italian study showed that premenopausal breast cancer patients who were given fenretinide, a drug related to vitamin A, had lower risk of developing a new cancer compared with women who did not receive the drug. The drug may have caused slightly more cancers, however, in the postmenopausal women who received it. The results, therefore, are not clear, and more research is needed before we can recommend the use of drugs such as this for breast cancer patients.

The Women's Intervention Nutrition Study (WINS) is testing the effect of a low-fat, high-fruit/vegetable diet on breast cancer recurrence and survival in a randomized clinical trial. Women are randomly assigned to the diet group or the control (usual diet) group. Results from this study will not be available for a few years, however.

Nutrition and diet are factors over which women can take control following a breast cancer diagnosis. Good general recommendations for a healthy diet that may reduce the risk of developing breast cancer or prevent its recurrence include:

- Reduce excess body fat through exercise and a healthy diet.
- Limit dietary fat to less than 30 percent of total calories.
- Eat a balanced diet with a good variety of nutrients and plenty of fiber—this means plenty of fruits and vegetables!
- If you drink alcohol, do so only in moderation. This means no more than two drinks per day—fewer is even better.

✐   Selective Estrogen Receptor Modulators

Tamoxifen belongs to a group of medications called selective estrogen receptor modulators, or SERMs. Tamoxifen has been tested in clinical trials in more than 36,000 women around the world. A combined analysis of these studies found that patients who took tamoxifen for five years had only half the chance of developing a second breast cancer compared with women who did not take tamoxifen. A recent study in 1,804 patients with ductal carcinoma in situ, a preinvasive cancer, found similar results. The risk of subsequent invasive breast cancer was reduced by 43 percent in women who took tamoxifen therapy. Since women who have had invasive or noninvasive breast cancer are at a higher than average risk of developing a second breast cancer, the prevention effects of tamoxifen should be considered in all breast cancer survivors. There are risks associated with tamoxifen use, including endometrial (uterine) cancer, blood clots, strokes, cataracts, hot flashes, and vaginal discharge. For women with invasive or preinvasive breast cancer, the prevention benefits of tamoxifen may very well outweigh its risks. You should talk with your oncologist or breast surgeon about whether tamoxifen is appropriate for you.

Raloxifene (Evista) is a newer selective estrogen receptor modulator, similar to tamoxifen. The major difference between tamoxifen and raloxifene is the effect on the endometrium. Raloxifene does not appear to stimulate the uterine lining and therefore should not lead to increased endometrial cancer. Raloxifene has been less studied with respect to breast cancer and currently is approved only for treatment of osteoporosis. The scientists who conducted the Tamoxifen Breast Cancer Prevention Trial are currently conducting a study comparing the breast cancer prevention effects of tamoxifen compared to raloxifene. The STAR trial (study of tamoxifen and raloxifene) is recruiting postmenopausal women with a higher than average risk of breast cancer, including women with a family history of breast cancer in close relatives, with some types of benign breast disease requiring biopsies, with reproductive and hormonal histories placing them at increased risk, or who are over sixty years of age. Until raloxifene has been further studied as a breast cancer treatment and prevention agent, its use cannot be recommended as a breast cancer reducing drug outside of the setting of a clinical trial.

Neither tamoxifen nor raloxifene is the perfect substitute for estrogen in the breast cancer patient. What we hope for in the near future is the "ideal SERM," which can treat hot flashes, help with memory, and decrease osteoporosis and heart disease while decreasing the risk of breast and uterine cancer.

Table 11.1. The Ideal SERM

SITE/SYMPTOM	IDEAL SERM	TAMOXIFEN	RALOXIFENE
Central nervous system	Full estrogen	Unknown	Unknown
Hot flashes	Full estrogen	Antiestrogen	Antiestrogen
Breast	Antiestrogen	Antiestrogen	Antiestrogen
Uterus	Antiestrogen	Estrogen/full estrogen	Antiestrogen
Cardiovascular	Full estrogen	Partial estrogen	Partial estrogen
Bones	Full estrogen	Partial estrogen	Partial estrogen

There are many unknowns in breast cancer treatment and survivorship, but we are learning more all the time. Meanwhile, you can act individually to reduce your risk of breast cancer recurrence through careful follow-up examinations, diet, exercise, and avoidance of unnecessary exposure to carcinogens. Some breast cancer survivors can participate in clinical trials. All of us can have hope for the future as we learn how to prevent breast cancer, how to improve our cure rates, and how to minimize the side effects and long-term consequences of breast cancer treatment.

Summary

- The most important factor in determining your prognosis, besides the type of cancer you have, is getting the best and most complete treatment possible. For most patients, some combination of surgery, radiation, chemotherapy, and hormone therapy is optimal.
- If you have had one breast cancer, your risk of a second breast cancer is higher than for women without breast cancer. Therefore, it is critically important that you get regular follow-

up screening, including mammograms, clinical breast exams, and breast self-examination. Your doctor will tell you how often you should be getting mammograms and clinical breast exams.

- Understanding your risk, from both genetics and other factors, can give you information about your risk for future breast or other cancers and can help you decide about risk reduction measures such as surgery and medications.
- Consider participating in a clinical trial. The extra monitoring and education you get in a trial, as well as possible access to new treatments, may improve your prognosis.
- Take care of your emotional side. Dealing with breast cancer drains your emotional and physical strength. Draw strength from your loved ones, friends, and community. Join a support group or find other breast cancer survivors with whom you can share your concerns and fears—and your successes.

12

Optimizing Overall Health After a Diagnosis of Breast Cancer

One in eight women in the United States will develop breast cancer in her lifetime, but only one in thirty will die of breast cancer. As many as 65 to 70 percent of women with breast cancer survive this disease. Heart disease, osteoporosis, and menopausal symptoms are major health problems for all women, including breast cancer survivors. Although cancer is understandably the number-one concern for women undergoing breast cancer treatment, it is important to work on maintaining and improving your overall health as part of an optimal breast cancer recovery program. In this chapter, we discuss the symptoms and adverse effects of the sudden menopause state often created by treatment for breast cancer. We extend the discussion to include dealing with menopause without estrogen, since most doctors recommend against estrogen replacement for breast cancer patients. We give tips for dealing with menopause symptoms including hot flashes, insomnia, vaginal and urinary problems, emotional problems, and sexuality issues. We also give some tips on protecting your bones and heart, as you could be more prone to osteoporosis and heart disease without estrogen.

After you have been treated for cancer, you have two ongoing health needs: breast cancer–related health issues and overall health issues. You should have regular general health checkups, with screening for other diseases and types of cancer appropriate for anyone your age. Women who have had breast cancer have a slightly higher risk of developing other cancers, including ovarian and colon cancer and a second breast cancer. With early detection, these cancers often can be controlled. Annual pelvic examinations and Pap smears should be part of your optimal health program. Colon cancer screening should start at age fifty, earlier if a relative has had colon cancer. Practice good health habits: A healthy diet and exercise and getting enough sleep all help you feel better and decrease your risk of developing other health problems. Work as a partner with your health care team and take an active role in optimizing your long-term health.

Menopause Without Estrogen

Many women undergoing chemotherapy or hormone therapy for breast cancer experience hormonal changes and menopausal symptoms. When hormonal therapy (such as tamoxifen) is a part of the breast cancer treatment plan, it can cause menopausal symptoms even in patients who went through menopause many years before. Some women experience hot flashes, sweating, sleep or mood disturbances, vaginal dryness, and sexual difficulties. Younger patients may experience early menopause due to chemotherapy drugs that can affect ovarian function. Menstrual periods may become irregular or stop completely during chemotherapy. Whether a woman's menstrual periods resume after chemotherapy is influenced by her age when she began her treatment. Menstrual periods are more likely to stop if you are in your forties or older with your first breast cancer treatment.

Many doctors have a serious concern about using estrogen replacement therapy in women with a prior diagnosis of breast cancer. It is not possible to know for sure if a woman harbors hidden breast cancer cells in her body that might be stimulated to grow in response to estrogen. Once you have developed one breast cancer, you are at increased risk of developing a second breast cancer, as long as you have remaining breast tissue. Estrogen may increase that risk. Because women rarely take estrogen after a diagnosis of breast cancer, we don't have much scientific information about the risks and benefits of estrogen therapy for breast cancer patients. There are no studies that show that estrogen is harmful, but there are no studies that definitely show that it is safe, either. Clinical trials are attempting to determine the true risks and benefits of estrogen in breast cancer survivors.

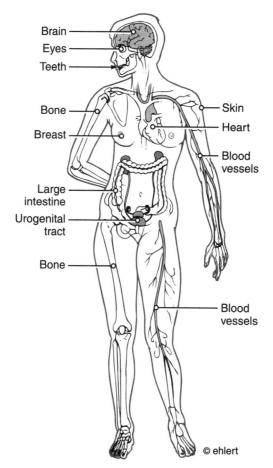

Figure 12.1. Estrogen affects most organs in the body.

Because breast cancer treatment often produces the sudden onset of menopause, women may struggle as they try to find ways to manage and deal with the associated side effects. Some breast cancer survivors suffer very severe symptoms of estrogen deficiency. The information provided below can help all breast cancer survivors manage symptoms related to menopause and optimize overall health.

Dealing with Hot Flashes

Blood vessels can become unstable in the amount of blood that they carry to the skin. This results in hot flashes and frequent awakening with night sweats. Here are some things that you can do lessen the severity and frequency of hot flashes.

- Examine triggers: strong emotions, caffeine, alcohol, cayenne or other spices, heavy or tight clothing, heat.
- Exercise: walk, swim, dance, pedal, or row twenty to thirty minutes each day.
- Sleep in a cool, well-ventilated room.
- Use fans.
- Wear clothes that "breathe," such as cotton or breathable synthetics, and dress in layers.
- Try deep, slow abdominal breathing, six to eight breaths per minute. Practice fifteen minutes each morning and evening. Use deep breathing when you feel the onset of a hot flash to lessen the intensity.
- Consider daily meditation, prayer, tai chi, or yoga.
- Eat food high in soy and phytoestrogens. (You should discuss this with your doctor first, as some doctors believe that phytoestrogens could actually make breast cancer worse in some patients.)

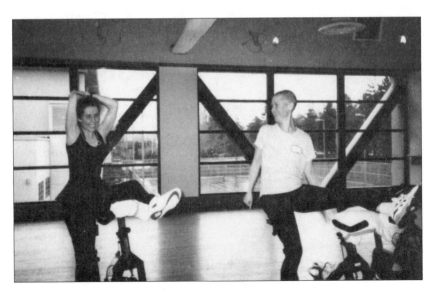

Indoor bike class called Heart Cycling at the Bellevue Athletic Club in Bellevue, Washington. Photo: Lisa Talbott.

- Find or create a support group.
- Try vitamin E, acupuncture, or botanicals (check with your health care provider before trying these).
- Stay well hydrated. Drink at least eight 8-ounce glasses of water each day.

Estrogen is clearly the most effective treatment for eliminating hot flashes, but this is not an option for most breast cancer survivors. If you have severe hot flashes, talk with your doctor about other medications, including clonidine (Catapres patch), bellergal, megestrol acetate (Megace), or antidepressants.

Osteoporosis

The bones begin to break down more rapidly when there is no estrogen to prevent calcium loss. This leads to loss of bone, a condition called osteopenia, and later to a more severe loss of bone called osteoporosis. With osteoporosis, women lose height as bones in the spine break or shrink in height. Painful fractures of the hip or spine may occur when a woman with osteoporosis falls. Hip fractures are a major cause of hospitalization and death in women as they age. Here are some tips for minimizing bone loss.

- Calcium can slow bone lose and decrease fractures. Take 1,500 milligrams of calcium per day from diet and/or supplements: 1,200 milligrams of calcium per day if you are premenopausal.
- Food sources of calcium include milk products, many green vegetables, and calcium-fortified orange juice and soy milk.
- Vitamin D helps calcium absorption and stimulates bone formation: 200–400 IU of vitamin D per day is advisable for all women.
- Drugs such as bisphosphonates (alendronate [Fosamax]), calcitonin, selective estrogen receptor modulators (such as raloxifene [Evista] and tamoxifen) can help reduce the rate of bone loss and osteoporosis.
- Avoid caffeine and tobacco, both of which can increase bone loss.

- Walking and muscle-building exercise are important in preventing bone loss and improving balance.

Preventing Heart Disease

Lack of estrogen speeds up the development of heart disease. Women begin to catch up with men in their risk of having a heart attack after they lose estrogen. Death from heart disease is about eight times more common than death due to breast cancer in older American women. There are several things that you can do to prevent heart disease.

- Exercise. Develop and maintain a routine with thirty minutes per day or more of moderate exercise. It can be ten to fifteen minutes at a time. Walk, climb stairs, bicycle, garden, dance, swim, row.
- Don't smoke.
- Eat a healthy low-fat diet. Include a wide variety of vegetables, fruits, and whole grains every day. Prepare without frying or adding extra oil. Use olive or canola oil when you do cook with oil. Avoid excess butter and margarine. Read the labels on your food products. Avoid items high in fat and cholesterol. Limit or avoid salt, cholesterol, and fat. Try to limit your diet to less than 20 grams of saturated fat per day.
- If you have high blood cholesterol levels despite a good diet, consider a cholesterol-lowering medication.
- If you have high blood pressure or diabetes, make sure these problems are well controlled.
- Have a self-calming practice (prayer, meditation, yoga, slow abdominal breathing).

Menopausal Insomnia

Hormonal changes as well as aging can influence sleep patterns. Many women experience insomnia during and following treatment for breast cancer. If you having trouble falling or staying asleep, you can try the following.

- Keep the room cool and well ventilated; 64 to 66 degrees is ideal.
- Wool blankets regulate skin and body temperature better than nylon or acrylic.
- Exercise daily.
- Avoid caffeine and excess alcohol in the evening.
- Avoid simple sugars (candy, cake, or cookies) at bedtime.
- Do not go to bed right after eating a meal, but do not go to bed feeling excessively hungry either.
- Take a warm shower or bath at bedtime or after waking during your sleep time.
- Try cereal and milk products at bedtime or after waking during your sleep time.
- Do not associate your bedroom with your workplace. Instead, think of it as your place for peace, relaxation, and sleep.
- Try to develop a routine of going to bed and getting up at the same times of day. If you have not fallen asleep after twenty to thirty minutes, get up and leave the bedroom.
- Avoid nicotine. Give up cigarettes.

Emotional Health: Dealing with Mood Swings, Depression, Anxiety, Fears, and Despair

Surgery, radiation therapy, chemotherapy, and hormonal therapy can cause intense psychological consequences. A significant number of breast cancer survivors have difficulty adapting to breast cancer diagnosis and treatment and experience disturbances in mood, body image, and self-worth. Disruptions in social, sexual, and family relationships can occur. Emotional distress related to fears of recurrence and death are not uncommon or abnormal. Recognizing this, and asking for help, is the first step on the road to emotional well-being.

Depression and anxiety are prominent feelings following a diagnosis of breast cancer. Studies have found that up to 40 percent of long-term breast cancer survivors felt depressed because of their breast cancer, and 64 percent had high anxiety. A lack of estrogen can contribute to the emotional aspect of breast cancer diagnosis, treatment, and recovery by causing the brain to function differently. This can result in depression, memory loss, mood swings, irritability, or a general sense of not feeling well. You can improve your emotional well-being with some of the following.

- Get involved with a support group or psychotherapy.
- Spend time reading favorite poetry or words of inspiration.
- Stay connected to your community and nourish your friendships.
- Have a self-calming practice (prayer, meditation, yoga, slow abdominal breathing).
- Find and practice outlets that renew your spirit and your tranquility.
- Avoid tranquilizers, if possible, as they can be habit-forming and can leave you feeling groggy when you are awake.

Urogenital Tract Atrophy

When ovarian production of estrogen stops or is significantly decreased, all areas of the body stimulated by estrogen undergo some change. The urogenital tract, which includes the bladder, uterus, and vagina, loses tissue in a process called atrophy. The vulva (external genital area) and vagina thin and become less moist. This causes symptoms of burning and pain when urinating, sudden loss of urine (incontinence), dryness and itching of the vagina, and sometimes pain during intercourse. There are several ways to decrease the severity and impact of these symptoms.

- Avoid chemical or mechanical irritants in the vaginal area. Wash with warm water and a soft cloth or your finger. Don't use soap or feminine wash products.
- Always wipe front to back.
- Apply a sparing amount of vitamin E oil to the external genital area (not into the vagina) to prevent wicking away of your natural moisture.
- When the area feels irritated or itchy, but your discharge is the same as always, try a small amount of lanolin cream to the external genital area (not into the vagina).

- Moisturizers or lubricants may be used in the vagina for comfort. Replens adheres to the vaginal wall and is intended to be used as a vaginal moisturizer, as opposed to a sexual lubricant. Try bacteriostatic water-soluble lubricants for intercourse or vaginal penetration. Examples are Astroglide, Slippery Stuff, Gyne-moisten, and K-Y.
- If the above suggestions fail, talk to your health care provider about using small amounts of estrogen in the vaginal area, such as a vaginal estrogen cream or the Estring. Any topical estrogen can be absorbed in small amounts into the bloodstream, so caution is advised in using this treatment approach.

Sexuality

Sexuality, self-esteem, and femininity are important issues that affect women undergoing treatment for breast cancer. You may notice decreased sex drive and pain with sexual intercourse. Your body image following breast cancer treatment may affect your feelings of sexuality. While undergoing breast cancer treatment you may be more focused on other issues, including your treatment and its side effects. Your partner may experience this as a withdrawal. Remember that you are both coping with a shift in roles as you adjust to many changes. You may have feelings of insecurity and guilt. Experiencing these difficult feelings is a normal part of the coping process. Allow yourself time to adapt to the changes in your body, self-image, and feelings about yourself, and to reestablish physical intimacy with your partner. The ability to feel pleasure from touching almost always remains. Nerves and muscles involved in the sensation of orgasm (climax) are not lost because of menopause. You can keep your sexual life alive during and after breast cancer treatment.

- Keep an open mind about different ways to feel sexual pleasure.
- Menopause may give you and your partner an opportunity to learn new ways to give and receive sexual pleasure.
- Strive to maintain open communication with your partner

about the changes that are taking place. Discussing your feelings with your partner and expressing your desire for physical affection is necessary for maintaining closeness.

- Take time to relax and become aroused. Be sensitive to your level of energy. If you are too tired at the end of the day, consider taking time with your partner in the morning or afternoon.
- Create an environment that enhances your sensuality and sexuality. Consider lighting, clothing, aromas, warmth or coolness.
- If sexual problems persist, be sure to talk to your health care provider and have a thorough pelvic exam.
- Therapy may help you and your partner develop better communication and reestablish your enjoyment of sexual intimacy.

Summary

- The majority of breast cancer patients can look forward to a long life after their diagnosis and treatment. This means that your health care should include care for all aspects of your health and well-being.
- Many breast cancer patients experience new or worsening menopausal symptoms. There are several home therapies that you can use to relieve these symptoms.
- Most doctors recommend that breast cancer patients limit their exposure to estrogen, which means not taking estrogen replacement therapy and using vaginal estrogen creams sparingly if at all.
- Osteoporosis and heart disease occur more often in postmenopausal women, but many lifestyle changes and medications can help to prevent these diseases.

13

Team Survivor

We are pleased to introduce you to Team Survivor in this chapter. We present the history, mission, and strategies of the Team Survivor programs. More important, we present personal testimonials of women who have made exercise an important part of their lives through their involvement with Team Survivor. We hope that you enjoy reading their stories as much as we have.

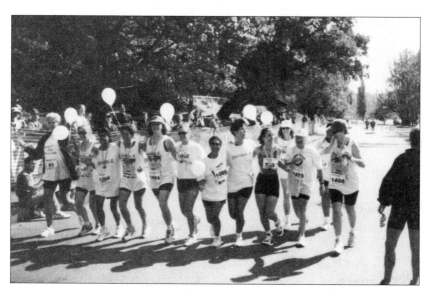

Team Survivor crossing the finish line at the Danskin Triathlon in Seattle

✐   The History of Team Survivor

During a swim in the Caribbean in 1995, professional triathlete Sally Edwards had an insight that would soon change the lives of many women around the country. She thought if breast cancer survivors could reach the summits of mountains, then they could certainly train and finish a triathlon. Sally conceived of the idea of creating "teams" of breast cancer survivors to participate in the Danskin Women's Triathlon Series. Her goal was to honor breast cancer survivors and build cancer awareness and visibility of the official race charity, the Susan G. Komen Breast Cancer Foundation. She brought her idea to Maggie Sullivan, VP of Sports Marketing at Danskin Inc., who agreed to support those teams and to help Sally create Team Survivor triathlon training programs in all six race cities. Breast cancer survivors together with their coaches, doctors, and other volunteers spread the word of this new innovative exercise program called Team Survivor throughout their communities. Women were encouraged to participate in the entire event, which included a half-mile swim, a twelve-mile bike ride, and a three-mile run. Many of the women had never even seen a triathlon, let alone participated in one. A number of women were in cancer treatment and chose to join the Walking Team or to do one event as part of a relay team. The local coaches created weekly swimming, biking, running, and walking groups to prepare women for these events. Sixty women participated in the first Danskin Team Survivor program in 1995. Today, as the national director of Danskin Team Survivor, Lisa Talbott continues to expand these training programs; there are expected to be more than 400 team members participating in the Year 2000 program!

During the weeks of training for the 1995 Danskin events, Lisa Talbott and team physician Dr. Julie Gralow met numerous women in Seattle who wanted to exercise but needed more support than the Danskin program could provide. Lisa and Julie decided to create year-round exercise programs that would give women with any type of cancer a safe place to recover physically from their treatments and surgeries. Together with the help of the University of Washington Cancer Center, they founded the nonprofit organization Team Survivor Northwest. This project was created with the enthusiasm and help of numerous volunteers from the cancer, medical, and fitness communities. It was designed to promote regular exercise, new and challenging physical goals, emotional and social support, and an emphasis on wellness. Over the next five years, Team Survivor Northwest helped other Team Survivor groups form around the United States. Currently, more than 3,000 women participate in Team Survivor exercise programs, educational classes, and fun fitness events in sixteen cities and nine states. The mission of Team Survivor is to encourage women cancer survivors to take an active role in their health and well being. Team Survivor USA, the national association of Team Survivor, is based in Texas and continues to support the growth of the Team Survivor wellness concept.

What Is Team Survivor?

Team Survivor promotes fitness by giving cancer survivors the support, skills, and knowledge needed to reach and maintain their health and fitness goals. Women who are actively undergoing chemotherapy or radiation treatment, recovering from surgery, affected by advanced disease, or dealing with survivorship issues can all benefit from Team Survivor programs. General physical health is promoted through weekly monitored exercise sessions; walking programs; and educational forums on health, exercise, and cancer, such as lymphedema, nutrition, alternative health, and stress management. Instructional clinics also teach skills needed to safely and successfully maintain activities such as swimming and biking. Monthly bike rides and hikes are organized, as well as special seasonal events including swimming, snowshoeing, and skiing, to which women are welcome to invite family or friends. Social and emotional support evolves from the camaraderie, encouragement, and communication involved in participating in activities with other women who share similar life experiences, attitudes, and goals. The structure of Team Survivor provides a unique opportunity for participants to benefit from and develop both physically and emotionally, while proceeding at an individual pace.

Team Survivor is open to all women with a past or present diagnosis of cancer. Participants range in age from twenty-five to eighty. Team Survivor attracts women who do not feel comfortable in traditional support groups or in other public exercise arenas. Participation in challenging and rewarding fitness events is a special component of Team Survivor. Many women facing a diagnosis of cancer need to prove to themselves and others that they are "okay." Most rethink the purpose, goals, and direction of their lives and make a commitment to experiencing and accomplishing things for which they never had time or never thought possible. Fitness challenges provide stimuli that encourage personal growth through succeeding at new and difficult experiences. Team Survivor encourages participation in local fitness events such as 5K walks/runs, triathlons, hiking, biking, and yoga events. Team Survivor members have climbed mountains, participated in 200-mile bike rides, competed in triathlons, and run marathons. Setting and achieving physical or health-related goals provide personal satisfaction and proof that life does exist after cancer.

Personal Testimonials of Team Survivor Members

Here are the stories of some Team Survivor members, all breast cancer survivors who used exercise as part of their treatment and recovery process. These women are of all ages, all stages of diagnosis, with differing fitness levels and athletic abilities. We find them to be an amazing and inspirational group of women, and we think you will, too.

Belinda's Story

The first time I was diagnosed with breast cancer was in 1989. I had a lumpectomy on my right breast. The lymph nodes that were removed were negative. I went through radiation and chemotherapy. I was teaching first grade at the time, and I continued working during my therapy. The doctors thought that they had caught my tumor in time. In 1994 I had a recurrence of the cancer. It had spread to my liver and bones. The doctor told me that the cancer was terminal and that I had one or two years to live. We began aggressive treatment. I developed congestive heart failure and could not have a planned stem cell transplant. I was put on tamoxifen when the chemotherapy failed. My heart ejection fraction (the heart's ability to pump) was severely reduced at 30 percent, and I was told this would not get better. My husband said that if I could exercise and strengthen my heart, maybe I would live long enough for there to be a new treatment. I started going on walks with my neighbor Tina

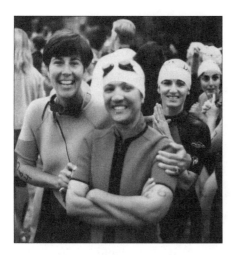

Belinda Ishem (right) with fellow team member and executive director of Team Survivor Northwest, Julia Cañas

and her dog. At first it took me forty-five minutes to walk a block. A few months later I could walk a mile in forty-five minutes!

One day, while looking through my mail, I found an invitation for cancer survivors. A few weeks later I went to a meeting of Team Survivor. The group was watching a video of a triathlon that they had completed. I was amazed. I remarked that there was no way I could do anything like that. A lady next to me asked me, "Why not?" I told her that I didn't have a bike. She said, "So get one." I said that I had not ridden since high school. She said, "So start riding." I said that I couldn't swim well enough. She said, "Practice." I said that I couldn't run. This lovely lady, Bonnie Wegner, said, "Walk."

I finished my first triathlon on August 19, 1996. I had just gone into remission. I finished two more triathlons in 1997 and 1998. They have been wonderful experiences for me. I have a bike, a cool helmet, an iron-man wet suit, and cross-training shoes. Tamoxifen has been replaced with anastrazole. I am still battling cancer—I will always have to fight. Every day I thank God for my life. I'm stage IV and still here. Who knew?

Bonnie's Story

I've always been active and semiconscious of what I ate, and yet here I was facing a diagnosis of breast cancer. I had to get my mind and body back into control. Two weeks after my mastectomy I felt I had to run, walk, or "whatever" a local seven-mile race. Shepherded by a friend, I completed it, no personal record in terms of time but a personal record in the sense of feeling my mind come back into control and joining the living. I continue running, but not with my prosthesis; I have enough spots to chafe without that. I was self-conscious without it, but I've had

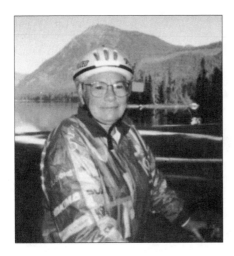

Bonnie Wegner enjoys cycling and encourages women to find the joys of bike riding.

other runners give me a thumbs-up "way to go" as they pass. I'm not fast, I just can last. I love long-distance bike rides and have ridden from Seattle to Maine twice. On one trip I got a small hole in my prosthesis and I was getting smaller on one side, so I patched the prosthesis with my tire patch kit! I still run, walk, swim, play tennis, and bike. After some hand repair surgery, I'll do another cross-country bike trip this fall.

Exercise has certainly been my lifesaver in putting my mind and body back together again. I can't begin to tell you about the depth of feeling between cancer survivors. We've been there, seen it all, and together we're finding our way.

Vibeke's Story

I'm thirty-eight years old and have been a diabetic since 1971. I moved from Denmark to the United States in October 1992. In Denmark I played in a badminton league with training and matches approximately ten hours per week, I bicycled back and forth to work (seven miles each way), and I jogged twice a week. Badminton is not a big sport in the United States, bicycling on the streets is dangerous, and somehow I did not get out jogging. So my exercise came to a screaming halt with my arrival in Seattle.

In August 1997, twenty pounds heavier, I was diagnosed with breast cancer. I received sixteen weeks of chemotherapy followed by mastectomy and lymph node removal. From my first day of chemotherapy I started walking, sometimes by myself, but mostly with my great husband and wonderful daughter (she was in a stroller). I knew that the exercise and fresh air would help me cope with the emotional thoughts that arise with the diagnosis of cancer. Walking was a good way of getting my mind cleared, and I was happy every time I could get up the hill near our house without breathing too hard. There was a little troll in my mind jumping up saying, "The cancer will not get me, I will beat it." The best conversations I ever had with my husband were on these walks—no telephones, no television, and no distraction from others. Everything looks nicer and clearer when walking. I changed to be partly vegetarian, dropped coffee, and ate more vitamins and flaxseed oil. The feeling of accomplishing something I believed in helped me deal with my cancer.

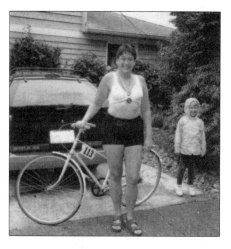

Vibecke Brinck following her first Danskin Triathlon, pictured with daughter, Mary

After my stitches were removed in December 1997 I needed to exercise my right arm, so besides the exercise schedule from the hospital, I started swimming in a pool at a fitness center. It was a little difficult in the beginning, but it helped me get the strength back in my arm very fast. From then on I continued with my swimming, and I starting bicycling in the fitness center and did some jogging, too. When I completed the Danskin triathlon in 1999 with my doctor at my side, I felt that we had helped defeat my cancer as we worked on getting to that finish line. I have just started a kick-boxing program once a week and am enjoying it. As soon as the snow arrives, you will find me skiing down the slopes. I am sure the exercise helped me through the cancer treatment and recovery. I am a true believer that keeping up my exercise with healthy eating habits will allow me to see my grandchildren one day.

Linda-Jo's Story

I have been exercising regularly with aerobics and weight training, three times a week, for about thirteen years. It's a big part of stress management for me. I was diagnosed in May 1998 with a 1.1-centimeter breast cancer. My surgery was on a Thursday—a lumpectomy and sentinel lymph node biopsy. I rested over the weekend and had my appointment for results the following Tuesday. Tuesday morning I went to the health club—only five days after surgery. I took it easy, but it felt so good to do the weights that I could and to dance in class to get rid of that invalid feeling. And to take my mind off what I might hear that afternoon. After the doctor said that everything had gone well (negative nodes and clear margins), my husband told him that I had gone to the club and asked him to tell me not to. The surgeon turned to me, congratulated me, and told me to go if I felt up to it.

I know that getting right back into exercise was part of how quickly I regained my arm mobility. Three weeks after surgery I was able to folk dance and let my partners twirl me with my arm stretched all the way up. It felt joyous! Next I underwent chemotherapy and radiation. I kept exercising all through treatment. I felt like it helped my body, my mind, and my spirit to keep going to the club. It was a great break from doing treatment things, a great release for tension, and a great source of satisfaction and pride that I could keep taking care of myself, of my muscles and the rest of my body, while I fought off the cancer.

I was thrilled to find Team Survivor. The first time I went, I received information about how much I could do, how to set sensible limits, and what to watch out for. I had been worried that with all the stress radiation and chemotherapy would put on my body, exercise would make it worse instead of better. I was reassured that I could get the benefits I wanted without hurting myself. I told my aerobics instructors what I was going through as I lowered my step in class, and they were helpful in adjusting intensity. People in my athletic club were a great cheering section as I worked through chemo. They were complimentary when I was working out bald and congratulatory as my hair grew back in. They even contributed more

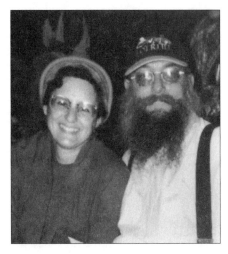

Linda-Jo Brooke and husband, Dane

than $400 to the Komen Foundation's Race for the Cure when I announced that I was going to do it.

Exercise gave me some sense of normalcy; my entire life was not about cancer. Even days when I could do only a light workout, I left the club feeling better. It took about five months for me to get completely back to the level of workouts I had been at before cancer. I am now on an even more intense weight-training program and am back to the same aerobic intensity as before. I am sure that continuing to exercise helped me to counteract and fight off the side effects of the chemotherapy. I could have gotten through cancer and treatment without exercise, but I am sure I would have been more uncomfortable and grumpy, and I would have gained weight.

Carol's Story

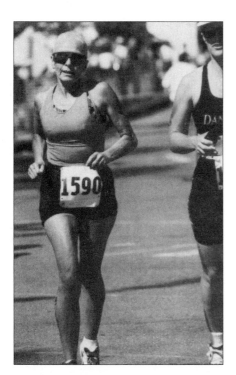

Carol Eaton (left) at one of her many triathlon races running with coach Michelle Kunzwiler

I am a sixty-four-year-old member of Team Survivor. This program fit right into my lifestyle of exercise that began even before I was diagnosed with breast cancer. When I was diagnosed with bilateral breast cancer in March 1997, I was stunned, like someone or something whacked my head. I was dizzy and disoriented. I was alone in the doctor's office that afternoon, so as I left the office I incorporated exercise into my reaction to my diagnosis. I was very, very sad. I took a long walk before I went to my car. The walk did not make me feel better about cancer, but it allowed me some time to think and grieve before I drove home.

Of course cancer changed

my life. Now my motto is to do the things I have always wanted to do NOW. During my chemotherapy treatment I did two triathlons because I thought I had better challenge myself some more now just in case next year I felt worse. As it turned out, doing those triathlons with the support of my family (especially my husband), Team Survivor, and my doctor benefited my mood and made me feel like I could beat this disease. Physically, somehow, I felt better, too. Now six days of exercise a week is a must for me. Most of the time I feel like I never had cancer. I continue to challenge myself so I can meet and beat life's barriers. Now every summer my husband and I bike up and down a mountain in Canada. It is a tough mountain bike ride for me. I never did that before my cancer diagnosis.

So, you see, challenging myself with new or more difficult exercise events helps me physically, mentally, and emotionally. I am in good health, physically fit, work at a challenging job, and have a "fighting" attitude.

Jeanne's Story

You don't have to be an athlete to enjoy exercise as part of your lifestyle. And you are never too old to begin. I began doing aerobics at age fifty-three. I was diagnosed with breast cancer in the summer of 1989, and immediately after surgery I continued aerobics in a limited way during the six weeks of radiation. Then I left on a planned trip to Papua New Guinea for four weeks of rather active travel. I felt great.

In 1995, a member of Team Survivor Northwest introduced me to some of their activities. I began cycling and learning bike care and attended Wednesday evening workouts. In 1997, Team Survivor introduced me to snowshoeing. I love the great exercise it provides and the

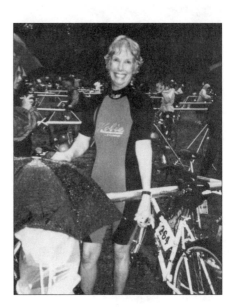

Jeanne Eaton (no relation to Carol Eaton) at the finish of a rainy Danskin race

beauty of the surroundings. In 1998, I began to train for the Danskin Women's Triathlon. Team Survivor provided us with a coach, training activities, schedules, and SUPPORT. It was a dark, rainy morning as I took off on the half-mile swim. It was as difficult as I expected, but I came out of the water to cheers and actually found the twelve-mile bike ride to be fun. Our ages were written on the back of our calves, and as the younger, stronger riders passed me and read the "68," they cheered me on. As I crossed the finish line with three other Team Survivor members, our arms on each other's shoulders, it was a great moment. I placed first in my age group (sixty-five to sixty-nine), but I must confess that I don't believe I had much competition. The important thing was that I finished AND I felt great afterward—that was my goal. The friends I have made through exercising have been a wonderful plus and have added much to my life in ways other than exercise.

Nina's Story

Exercise has always been a part of my life, but I took it for granted until I was diagnosed with breast cancer at age forty-nine in 1994. I was deter-mined to keep up my running during the ensuing seven months of treat-ment, although it became very difficult toward the end. Still, it gave me some continuity and a great deal of peace of mind. During the following year of recovery, I found myself deeply immersed in my exercise rou-tine. Suddenly, I had become afflicted with the "if I feel good and I look good I can't possibly be sick" syndrome. Support from my family and friends and Team Survivor Northwest both motivated and inspired me. Within three years, I had com-pleted three triathlons and a 200-mile bike ride—and I even jumped out of a plane! I have

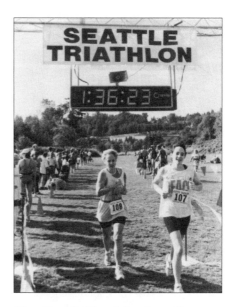

Nina Fogg (left) and daughter, Cara Holloway. Photo: Envirosports.

never felt better. Exercise has become both a physical and mental healing for me. It helps me keep a positive perspective on life and allows me to face each day with a healthy attitude. I am definitely a stronger person for what I have been through. I frequently tell cancer patients, "You will be the same person, only different—and maybe even better." I know I am.

Mary's Story

Physical activity and being outdoors in nature have always been a part of my life and who I am. When I was diagnosed with stage II breast cancer at age thirty-five, exercise became a major part of my healing. Two months into my chemotherapy I became a charter member of Team Survivor Northwest, a positive, friendly, and inspiring group of female cancer survivors. Meeting as strangers, we soon became fast friends bonded together by our common experience of cancer. It was my support group, combining physical activity and an atmosphere of unconditional acceptance. When I moved to Colorado, I had to leave my friends behind, but they will forever be in my heart and a continuing part of my life.

Seeing the importance and need for a similar group in Colorado, I established Rocky Mountain Team Survivor, which is now my pet project in addition to my "other job" as an oncology nurse. I have seen how women realize their physical, emotional, and inner strength by achieving goals they never thought they could achieve. I've experienced the connectedness that exists between women who share an experience of living with and through cancer, regaining their strength, their bodies, their lives. My dream is to continue to support, encourage, and challenge women cancer survivors with love. My future goal is to climb Mt. Kilimanjaro to

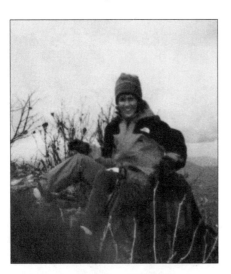

Mary Berg in her favorite place, the mountains. "Live well—laugh often—love much."

raise funds for breast cancer research. It's a natural fit: me, the outdoors, encouraging others, and experiencing life with love.

Joan's Story

In 1997, at the age of forty-nine, I was diagnosed with both ovarian and breast cancer. I was terrified. I had endless questions, and there were very few answers. I felt as though my body had let me down, and the treatments and surgeries further eroded my self-image. I was blessed to

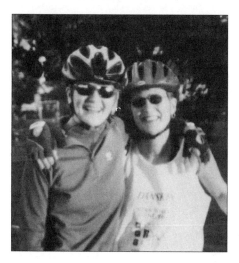

Joan McAree (right) and sister, Jean Christ

have emotional support from family and friends—my twin sister gave me strength and courage as I faced each medical test and treatment with her by my side. This outpouring of love and positive energy lifted my spirits and inspired me to focus on healing and wellness.

Following surgery I regained my stamina through exercise. As my physical strength increased, my positive outlook increased as well. I joined Team Survivor Northwest and was inspired and motivated by the camaraderie of fellow survivors. Through their support, I was empowered to raise my exercise and fitness goals to new levels. To celebrate the completion of chemotherapy, I participated in the Susan G. Komen Breast Cancer Foundation's Race for the Cure. One year later I entered my first triathlon. With the help of Team Survivor, I crossed the finish line as a strong and confident athlete! Being a member of Team Survivor reaffirms the importance fitness and exercise play in maintaining my healthy and positive outlook.

Sharon's Story

First, I must admit I am a competitive, determined, and motivated person. I was the top-ranked forty-to-forty-four-year-old female triathlete in the South/Midwest region for the 1998 season. I was on top of the world, in peak shape, and leading a healthier life than I ever had. Six days later I was diagnosed with breast cancer. I had a lumpectomy with sentinal node biopsy surgery.

The next weekend I was riding my bike, and a week later doing a track workout. I just pushed myself to do what I could. I found I could still do a lot. I would leave radiation and

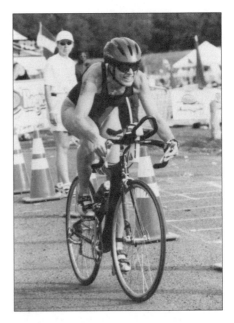

Sharon Rector crossing finish line.
Photo: Patsy Sutherland/
Peacockphoto.com.

go swimming or running. I didn't stop; I just slowed down. I found I could still place in my age division, although I was slower. Two and a half weeks into radiation treatment I won my age division at a challenging duathalon known for its harsh weather conditions. Then two weeks following the completion of radiation I did a Race for the Cure 5K run. I was the first survivor across the finish line and second in my age division. It helped ease some of the anger I had about getting the disease.

By far, the most comprehensive treatment I have found since my diagnosis has been Team Survivor Austin. As I already had a fairly high, intense training program, I joined Team Survivor for the emotional support and companionship found with the other women cancer survivors interested in fitness and health. The team helps me maintain a healthy balance in my life and makes each time I train and race count more. My present goal is to train and race as a visible cancer survivor to let other women cancer survivors know anything is possible. When Lance Armstrong, a testicular cancer survivor, won the 1999 Tour de France, he said it all: "If you ever get a second chance in life, you've got to go all the way."

Judith's Story

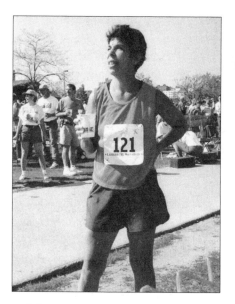

Judith Ormond has fallen in love with running and uses her experience to encourage women with cancer in the Milwaukee area to stay active and exercise.

I had always considered myself to be more of a sloth than an athlete. I am short and have heavy legs. As a child, I hated gym. I used to think that I was in total control of my body— that is, until two months before my fiftieth birthday, two months before my long-planned, age-defying bicycle trip through Bali. In May of 1996, I went to a surgeon for a needle biopsy on a suspicious lump on my left breast. It was cancer. Surgery was at the end of May. In July, immediately following my second chemo and with the hesitant blessings of my doctors, I was off on my bicycling trip in Bali. I was feeling fit and fortunate to be on an island of sacred mountains, an island of warm, life-embracing people. Bali was so far away from cancer. Radiation began on Labor Day. I knew about the fatigue effects of radiation, but it wasn't going to happen to me because I was fit. I planned to conquer the fatigue. Prior to my daily morning appointments, I ran four miles. By the end of seven weeks, I was exhausted. For a year, I could barely move.

In the spring of 1998, I read about the Susan G. Komen Race for the Cure in Madison. It was 5 kilometers. I could barely run half a mile. I hired a personal trainer. I was ready to take control again. By the end of May, I ran Race for the Cure. At that moment, my self-image transformed from one of little confidence to one of guts and glory. It was as though Cinderella's godmother had touched me with her magic wand. My life, my body were mine once again. I cried with joy, with relief, and with the realization that I had once again taken control. I had empowered myself. I beat my cancer!

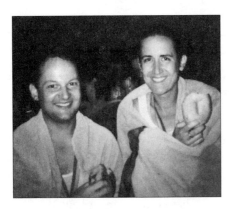

Karen Van Kirk and husband, Andy, staying warm at the finish of the Los Angeles marathon

Karen V.'s Story

The first few hours after I learned that I had been diagnosed with breast cancer were a jumble of phone calls, confusion, and emotion. One of the first clear and constructive thoughts I had during that time, however, was that continuing my running routine was likely to be a big help in coping with whatever was ahead. During the next few weeks of uncertainty and fear, I found that I felt happy, almost giddy, when I went out for a run. My running represented a part of my life that I could control. No matter what I was to learn about my prognosis over the coming weeks, there would still be a part of my life that I could define and manage strictly for myself.

As I went through the treatment course, my energy level dropped significantly, and the bulk of my running shifted to walking. Despite a good prognosis, I was emotionally fragile, and I experienced every feeling very deeply. Knowing that my walks gave me uninterrupted time for introspection made this barrage of feelings much less intimidating. A month after my treatment was complete, I set out with my husband, Andy, for one of our favorite runs, on a trail near the Connecticut River and the Dartmouth College campus. It was the longest run I had taken since my diagnosis, and I surprised myself a bit with my stamina. During the last half mile, a steep and rocky hill, I recognized a different type of fatigue from what I had been experiencing over the previous few months. "This fatigue isn't about the cancer," I told myself, "this fatigue is about being an athlete and training and *not hanging back from this hill.*" I gave a quiet "thank you" to the runner in me, recognizing how important she had been as I struggled with the feelings surrounding my cancer and looking forward to an ongoing recovery process where I continued to feel strong and in control of my body and my health.

Kathy's Story

As I was growing up, exercise had always been a part of my life. I played competitive tennis and softball and also enjoyed biking, swimming, golfing, and skiing. In college, I took up canoeing and tried cross-country skiing. Little did I realize that a decade later, this exercise would help me cope and survive.

In June of 1989, my worst fear had come to be: I had cancer and would have to undergo chemotherapy. I thought my life was over, because at that time, I had never known anyone who had survived chemotherapy,

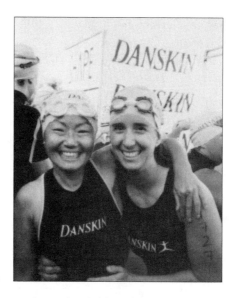

Kathy Nishizaki (left) with coach Lisa Talbott at the start of the Danskin Women's Triathlon in San Jose, California

let alone exercised while on chemo. This was a devastating thought, but my oncologist told me that I would still be able to live a normal life, though I might have to slow down. I was able to exercise daily, work full time, and continue to play softball and tennis.

Five years later, I had a heartbreaking recurrence and was told I would benefit from a bone marrow transplant. They told me I would probably be off work between six and eight months and would have to take it very easy. I was able to return to work within six weeks after the transplant—this I attributed to being in a somewhat good physical condition. I was happy to be on the road to recovery, but I continued to coddle myself because I was afraid to do anything too strenuous.

Seven months after the transplant, I heard about a women's triathlon where they had a program for women cancer survivors. I decided this would help me to start my "new life," and I joined the program, Team Survivor. I set a goal to try to run the 3.1-mile run without stopping—this alone would be a major accomplishment. Because I had not swum or biked in years. I decided to forgo the swimming and biking and to concentrate on the run. On race day, I decided to go ahead and do the swim accompanied by my coach. Although I hadn't trained for this part of the race, I just felt so empowered by all the women and support I was feeling that I went for it. Much to my amazement, I finished the swim and ran the entire 3.1 miles without stopping or walking! Thus began my "new life" and my road to recovery. Through exercise, the support of friends, family, the medical community, and God, I was able to accomplish something beyond my wildest dreams. The best part was that I was still intact after that first triathlon, and I am alive today to tell the story. With help, I was able to go beyond my limits. With this help, I am able to SURVIVE.

Susan's Story

When I was diagnosed with breast cancer in 1988, my parents asked if they could get me something that would help with my treatment and recovery. I called back the next day to ask for a six-month membership at a local health club so that I could swim. I was always active but never involved much in organized sports. I loved swimming when I was young because it helped a shy, somewhat gangly girl feel powerful and graceful.

As I grew older, I also appreciated that swimming focused and calmed me, much like meditation. For all of these reasons, I knew that I wanted to swim through radiation and chemotherapy and whatever followed—to help me feel powerful, graceful, focused, and calm—through a period during which I might otherwise feel powerless, ugly, and anxious. And so I swam, daily, through the aftermath of surgery, through skin-burning radiation, and through weary months of chemotherapy. Of all the habits that I tried to change, adopt, or

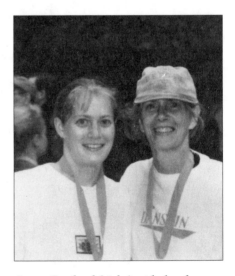

Susan Stockard (right) with daughter, Melissa, who first encouraged Susan to use sports to celebrate her ten-year anniversary of being cancer free

keep after the diagnosis of breast cancer, sticking to a regular exercise routine is the one that remains eleven years later.

In August 1997, my daughter called with an offer that I ultimately couldn't refuse: How would I like to come to Seattle in August 1998 to celebrate my tenth anniversary postcancer by participating in the Danskin Triathlon with her? Having a goal, working on it for a year, and achieving it was a thrill. Doing it with my daughter put it over the top. All my life, physical activity and exercise have helped my confidence and sense of well-being. By continuing to exercise, I continue to see myself as healthy.

Recently I was filling out a questionnaire that asked, "What comes first to mind when asked to describe yourself?" The first thing that came to mind was, "I am athletic." Only secondarily did I think, "Oh, and I had breast cancer."

Gail's Story

"The big one is malignant, and the little one is suspicious." Those eleven words that were said to me three years ago changed my life forever. I was

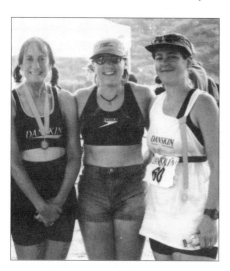

Gail DeRoy (left) with coach Andre Allaire (center) and friend and training partner Christine Bain (right), at the finish of her first Danskin Triathlon in Wrentham, Massachusetts

angry. It was bad enough that the mammograms didn't show it when it was small (dense tissue), but it seemed to happen at a time in my life when I didn't have time for cancer. I had a six-year-old at home, a full-time job, and activities I enjoyed doing. But life is not fair. I dropped everything and faced all that modern medicine had to offer me, including a mastectomy, chemotherapy, and reconstruction surgery. Three years later I am one happy woman. The reconstruction surgery, which included a "TRAM-flap" and implants, is natural and beautiful. I have embraced a very healthy lifestyle including a good diet and lots of aerobic exercise. I have entered and completed several triathlons in my area. I help other women survivors get back into shape and motivate others to get fit and healthy. I can do things today at forty-six I could not do at twenty-six! It is a very uplifting, empowering feeling, and most of all fun! I hope to continue helping other women face the demon and go on. Through exercise and feeling whole again, anyone can actually come out on top. Cancer does not have to be doom and gloom.

Karen H.'s Story

My original diagnosis of breast cancer came in 1993, when I was forty years old. Even though I had a family history, this was the last thing that I thought would happen to me. Yet here I was, about to be mutilated and poisoned to treat this insidious disease. I was grasping at whatever I could to help me maintain some sort of balance and control in my life. I was reading everything I could, attending a support group, trying complementary therapies, and getting my exercise. For me, exercise was my stabilizing factor. I was able to work out all during my chemo, just not at the same intensity. Hallelujah! When I completed my treatment, I was sure that I wouldn't have to deal with breast cancer again. I worked hard to regain my previous physical condition and felt great, and yes, I was still racing my bike!

But then the word that we all dread, "recurrence," came into my life. Four and one half years out from my diagnosis, I felt some ominous lymph nodes in my neck and a tiny spot of point tenderness on my sternum. As completely unbelievable as this was to me, I now had metastatic breast cancer. I chose to act as aggressively as possible with my treatment and elected to do a stem cell transplant. The odds given to me were that I had a 20 percent

Karen Hornbostel (right) with her mother, Lena

chance to survive five years after the transplant. Well, the way I thought of that was through a bike race. I thought of being on the start line of a race with 100 women and I needed to be in the top twenty at the finish. I realized that I could do that!

The stem cell transplant was a humbling experience. I hit a brief but intense depression during this period and contemplated medication for the depression. I decided to wait as I began to exercise again, and as soon as I got back into my regular routine, the depression quickly subsided. I again realized what a powerful tool exercise was for me. My recovery from the stem cell transplant has been slow, but I have been able to see gradual improvement. I'm able to train hard again, just not very fast, and I'm feeling great doing it! My competitive spirit is still there, and I'm looking forward to participating in a few bike races this year.

Whether cancer gets me in one year, twenty years, or not at all, I'm going to keep on living fully and appreciating everything I can. I also believe that it is imperative to stay as healthy and strong as possible, so that if I do have to face cancer again, I can give myself a better chance to survive the next round of treatment. Clearly, exercise has given me a sense of control and power over this disease and offers me hope that I will survive for many years to come.

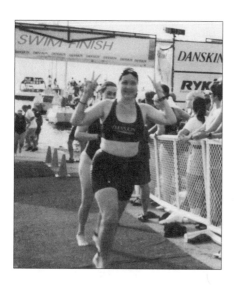

Carla Felsted finishing the swim on her fifth Danskin Triathlon in Austin, Texas. Photo: Lisa Talbott.

Carla's Story

Six weeks after my bilateral mastectomy and reconstruction, I suffered a triple ankle fracture. It was like getting up after one truck hit me, only to be hit by another. Perhaps that's what it took to get my attention, to make me stop and think about where my life was going and how I had not been taking care of myself. I had been a slender, active teenager and continued to exercise and enjoy the outdoors into my thirties. But a sedentary lifestyle and a typical, too-fat American diet had taken over. Early menopause had brought extra pounds and lethargy. Now I had a real wake-up call.

After recovering from the ankle repair surgery, I began to walk in my neighborhood. I found out about a water exercise program for cancer survivors. There I found not just physical recovery, but camaraderie with other survivors. In 1995, I was proud to walk the 5K portion of the Austin Danskin Triathlon with Team Survivor. My teammates challenged and inspired me. Along with the physical recovery came emotional healing, too. I conquered a great deal of fear and self-doubt, largely with the support of my training partners and the Team Survivor coaches, but also from friends and family. I now exercise four to five times a week, with my husband, a long-time friend, and my Team Survivor buddies. People I have not seen in several years say I look younger. That may be mainly flattery, but I do know I look and feel much healthier than I did seven years ago!

Colleen's Story

In my youth, I had never really excelled in sports, but I had always enjoyed physical exercise. I became interested in solo or group activities such as biking, hiking, camping, and swimming. My first date with my husband was to try cross-country skiing. These activities kept my physical performance in good shape.

When I received a call to come back for some repeat views of my annual mammogram, I wasn't worried because I couldn't feel any lumps and thought the doctor was being overly cautious since my mother had died from breast cancer. When the mammogram was repeated, a biopsy was recommended to evaluate some new calcifications. We discussed a date for the procedure. My response was, "I have a bike trip that I've been training for and unless it's a life-or-death

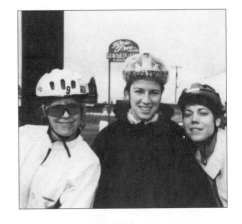

Colleen Zakar (left) with Donna and Porter of 2 Chicks, Two Bikes, One Cause Foundation, an organization dedicated to breast cancer awareness and support for younger women

situation. I would rather do the biopsy after the ride." The surgeon placed me on the schedule after my ride. I really felt it was important to do the bike ride. If it wasn't cancer, it seemed a waste to miss a good ride that I had trained for. If it was cancer, then I felt it was even more important to do the ride first and then go through the biopsy.

I did the ride in Eastern Washington and Idaho with friends and appreciated every moment. As I rode along a river I saw an eagle, enjoyed the beautiful colors of fall, and felt very thankful that I could be cycling in such lovely country. I returned home and went in for my biopsy and found out that I indeed had breast cancer. I truly felt the cycling I had done the previous week had helped put my mind in the right place to tolerate what I needed to do. I was able to relax by just visualizing where I had recently been and reminded myself that I could get through a tough day and could mentally place myself along the river in the sunshine again. The next few weeks were filled with appointments and making treatment decisions. I felt very thankful that I could rely on my "cycling escapes" to relax and rejuvenate.

Edree's Story

I do not call myself a breast cancer survivor. My adventure with inflammatory breast cancer lasted from January 1997 through October of the same year. That is ten months out of my fifty-two years of living. Although it was significant and extremely challenging, I won't define my life by that one experience. After I was diagnosed, someone gave me a copy of a famous book about breast cancer. In it, I found two lines on the type of breast cancer I was facing. The first line said that it was a rare type representing about 1 percent of the women

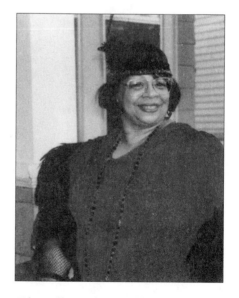

Edree Allen-Agbro danced for years for fun but now uses her love of dancing to also stay fit.

who had breast cancer. The second line informed me that the usual prognosis was about eighteen months. I threw the book away. I decided it was not good for my immune system to read such a thing! I also decided that I would make having minority status translate into a good thing again.

During treatment, I used every resource in my power to help me through. Many people prayed for me. I used my skills as a hypnotist to visualize. I listened to tapes. I cried. I prayed. I made love. I danced and laughed. I took complete charge. And I surrendered. During that time, I truly understood that I had 100 percent control over my destiny—and I had none. Now I am aiming for optimum health. I still have weight to release and habits not completely changed. I eat healthier, walk when it's warm, and dance as much as I can. Breast cancer made me even more determined to live life fully. I only have about forty-eight years left and I'm going to go through them. I'm actually going to have each and every experience of my life.

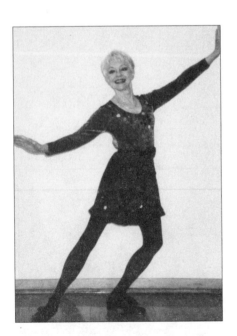

Lois Rathvon-McCarter continues to teach dance to people of all ages and stays fit dancing and performing with her dance troop, Swinging at Seventy. Photo: Doris Davis.

Lois's Story

I was over sixty and recently resigned as chair of a dance department when I was diagnosed with breast cancer and subsequently had a mastectomy. I continued to teach dance classes but became increasingly interested in movement and body awareness as they related to the healing process and one's general health. Significantly, my path crossed with Judy Ellis, a physical therapist and breast cancer survivor who had similar concerns. With a goal of assisting women to regain personal power and control following cancer treatment, we developed a movement awareness class for cancer survivors.

Based on dance and exercise, these classes help participants understand their physical body, which in turn enables them to realize that one has movement choices as well as mental choices. Deepak Chopra writes in *Ageless Body, Timeless Mind* that we are of three ages: chronological, biological, and psychological. We cannot change our chronological age, but we can slow and/or reverse our biological and psychological age.

Swinging at Seventy, a tap dance trio of which I am a member, believes that dancing is good for both body and spirit. Our program helps people in our age group realize that physical activity is an age-reversal process. We also hope others approaching the senior years will recognize the long-term health benefits of physical and mental challenge. Adaptability seems to be the key. Dance, in the broadest sense, is the best way to maintain both physical and mental adaptability.

Nancy's Story

I don't like exercise, and having the opportunity to experience breast cancer has not changed my feeling about this. I do work a little harder at trying to enjoy doing the things that will improve my physical health, but exercise for me is precisely that—work. Exercise seems to break up an otherwise wonderful day! I do therapeutic exercise for my bad knees and can honestly say that I have not missed a day of my lymphedema exercises. My motivation has everything to do with improving my ability to do other physical activity I love, such as leatherwork and playing with my dogs. I know about keeping a positive attitude—cancer has taught me that—but I can't seem to wrap my mind around sweating and breathing really hard as fun. I

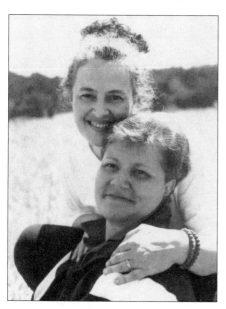

Nancy White (bottom) with partner, Heather, enjoy time at the coast, golfing, and being together. Photo: Campiche Studios.

have found some things that I truly love to do, such as in-line skating and riding my motorcycle. Most recently I have fallen in with golf. I do not do these things to lose weight or increase my fitness. I do these things for the pleasure of doing them. These activities help me feel whole, happy, and alive.

Thank you to all the women who shared their stories in this book and who share their stories with their doctors and other healers, fellow survivors, and people they meet every day who want to know more about cancer and exercise. There are

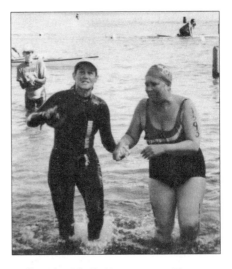

Sally Edwards (left) supports a Team Survivor member as she finishes the swim of her first triathlon. Photo: Lisa Talbott.

hundreds of incredible Team Survivor stories that have inspired women to take control of their health and keep faith in their bodies with exercise.

To join a Team Survivor program in your area, contact Team Survivor USA at www.teamsurvivor.org. Most Team Survivor programs are supported by volunteer efforts. What better way to stay in shape than to volunteer for a fitness organization like Team Survivor? You do not need to be a cancer survivor to volunteer for these programs. (See Appendix B for a Team Survivor group in your area.)

Summary

- Team Survivor is a health and fitness resource for women affected by cancer in all stages of treatment, recovery, and survivorship.
- Team Survivor promotes fitness by giving cancer survivors the support, skills, and knowledge needed to reach and maintain their health and fitness goals.

14

Develop a Health-Promoting Exercise Plan

Women who do aerobic exercise regularly at moderate to high intensity levels have a lower risk of developing breast cancer compared with more sedentary women. From the scientific evidence collected so far, we believe that daily aerobic exercise throughout your lifetime is important in reducing risk for breast cancer. We describe in this chapter the components of an aerobic exercise program, including frequency, duration, and intensity. We provide exercise guidelines to help you determine the appropriate intensity and amount of exercise to match your activity level and fitness goals. We provide some sample exercise programs for women wanting to reduce their risk for breast cancer as well as for breast cancer patients and survivors. We hope that this chapter will give you some basic building blocks for starting and maintaining a healthy exercise program for life!

In some epidemiological studies, a half hour per day on average was associated with a reduced risk for breast cancer, while in other studies it took an hour per day to provide the greatest reduction in risk. The epidemiological studies were all limited, however, because they were able to determine only the effects of exercises that the women had commonly done in the past. For example, if the women were most commonly doing popular activities such as walking, swimming, golf, and tennis, then those are the only activities about which the study can have findings. In all of the studies, too few women were doing those more vigorous exercises to allow the researchers to look at the individual exercise's effects on breast cancer risk. The researchers, therefore, summed all of the exercises into a small number of categories according to how intense they usually are for an average person. For this reason, we do not know if any particular exercise is more protective than another.

In giving our recommendations for the types of exercise that may reduce risk of breast cancer, therefore, we are making a leap of faith. We assume that the observed effect of exercise is real, that is, it is not due to something else that is different about exercisers, such as their diet. Second, we assume that everyone who does an exercise puts the same amount of energy into the exercise. We rely on the study participants to recall and report accurately the types and amounts of exercise they did currently and in the past. Finally, we assume that increasing exercise is a good thing for breast health. Given the assumptions, we are making the following recommendations.

For most women, the main goal for exercise and breast health is to avoid gains in fat mass with aging. As you exercise and become more fit, your muscle mass increases and your metabolism increases as a result. When measuring your body fat, also be sure to pay attention to how much muscle you are maintaining. It is easy to misinterpret your "percent body fat." Just by increasing your amount of muscle mass, you won't necessarily decrease the *amount* of fat on your body, but you will decrease your *percent* body fat. However, in terms of breast health, it is important also to keep a low amount of body fat.

Let's take the example of Joan. Joan is forty years old. She is 5' 2" and weighs 150 pounds. Her body mass index, or BMI, is 28.4. (For optimum health your BMI should be less than 25. See Appendix A.) Her lean mass is 99 pounds and her fat mass is 51 pounds. Her percent body fat therefore is $51 \div 150$ or 34 percent. She took up strength training for six months, and gained 10 pounds of muscle and no pounds of fat, so her new muscle mass is 109 pounds. Her new percent body fat is $51 \div 160$ or 32 percent. But her fat mass has stayed the same at 51 pounds. That fat tissue may still be making a lot of estrogen, so her breast health may not be improved compared to before she started strength training. If she is careful not to increase calories beyond what she ate when she started strength training, her larger muscles may start burning up some of her stored fat, so over the course of the next year she may lose some of the fat mass. If she adds an aerobic exercise program to optimize her rate of losing fat, she will speed up the rate of fat burning and will lose more fat.

If she loses 10 pounds of fat now, even though she has gained 10 pounds of muscle, her weight stays stable at 150. However, her fat weight will drop from 51 to 41 pounds, and her new percent body fat will be only 41÷150 or 27 percent! This percent body fat is much closer to what doctors recommend for good health for women.

There are many enjoyable exercises that you can do to avoid gaining fat and to lower the body fat you have. In general, higher-intensity exercise burns more body fat per hour than does lower-intensity exercise, as long as you do not exercise at too high an intensity (i.e., don't go above 85 percent of your maximum heart rate). Research indicates that to reduce risk for breast cancer, exercise must:

- Be aerobic. This means that you need to exercise above 50 percent of your maximum heart rate for all of the session, and at 65–85 percent of your maximum heart rate for most of the session. We describe how to determine these heart rate levels below.
- Cause sweating. If you sweat, it is more likely that your exercise is aerobic.
- Be done most days (ideally four to six days per week).
- Be done for a total of four or more hours per week.

Many types of exercise fit these criteria. Table 14.1 shows exercises you might try, along with the number of calories burned per hour. (See Appendix A for a more complete list of exercises.)

Table 14.1. Exercise and Calories Burned

EXERCISE	APPROXIMATE CALORIES BURNED (PER HOUR)*
Fast bicycling (14–16 miles per hour)	600
Running (5 miles per hour)	475
Singles tennis	475
Cross-country skiing (4–5 miles per hour)	475
Rowing (moderate, 4–6 miles per hour)	400
Jogging	400
Stationary bicycling (moderate, 150 watts)	400

* For a woman who weighs about 130 pounds.

EXERCISE	APPROXIMATE CALORIES BURNED (PER HOUR)*
Aerobic dancing	350
Stair-stepping machines	350
Brisk walking (3.5 miles per hour)	200
Golf (using motorized cart)	200

* For a woman who weighs about 130 pounds.

The amount of time you need to spend exercising depends on several things. First, if you need to lose extra fat mass, you should exercise often and for longer duration to mobilize and burn off the fat. You may also need to restrict calories somewhat. Second, the amount of exercise depends on your age, current weight, level of physical fitness, current health, and previous history of exercise and sports. Adding strength training, as we describe in Chapter 18, will help to speed up this process of fat loss, as it increases your fat-burning muscle mass. To devise an exercise plan that works for your schedule, needs, fitness level, and goals, consider the three key exercise components: frequency, duration, and intensity. Each workout is based on these three components, and the success of your overall personal plan is driven by how well you balance them.

Exercise Frequency

The number of times a day or week that you exercise is the frequency. This is one of the best places to start to monitor your progress and commitment to exercise. For new exercisers it is the most important component to monitor. Even for people already exercising, if your goal is regular exercise, then making sure you exercise often is the best way to build the exercise habit. Women sometimes choose to exercise more than once a day. This is helpful for women with busy schedules who for one reason or another need shorter bouts of exercise. In this situation, you would exercise twice a day for thirty minutes rather than once a day for an hour. What matters is the total time that you are exercising. Women who fatigue easily find it less tiring to do shorter amounts of exercise (say, ten minutes) two or three times a day to manage their fatigue. Sometimes an injury hurts less and heals quicker with shorter, more frequent exercise sessions. Beware of setting your goal to exercise every day if you are currently not exercising even once a week. It is unrealistic to change immediately from doing no workouts in a week to doing seven. Setting attainable frequency goals allows you to be successful.

Exercise Duration

The amount of time you spend in an exercise session is the duration. You should start with a comfortable length of exercise that keeps you feeling energized afterward. At first, it is best to start with a short exercise session. Exercising too long early on in your program may lead to frustration and fatigue. Some activities may require long duration, such as a half-day golf game or an hour-long aerobics class. Other activities can be done in several bursts throughout the day such as walking or stair climbing. For cardiovascular health most doctors recommend exercising for at least twenty to thirty minutes at a time at a moderate to high intensity level. To maintain fitness, several ten-minute bursts of exercise may be sufficient if the daily total is at least thirty to forty-five minutes. For weight loss and maintenance of low body fat, several shorter bursts of exercise may be sufficient if the daily total is at least forty-five minutes. Duration may also be gauged by an injury. For example, a knee may begin to hurt only if you run more than thirty minutes at one time.

Exercise Intensity

Intensity is how hard you exercise. This can be objectively measured by taking your heart rate or subjectively by estimating your perceived exertion. Your intensity increases when you do hills on a run or raise the gears on your bike. Your heart rate is the best way to monitor the intensity of your workout. Some exercises require high intensity to accomplish their goals. Other exercises can be done at medium or low intensity. For example, if you are somewhat fit, walking can be a stroll (low intensity), a moderately fast walk at 3.5 miles per hour (moderate intensity), or a speed-walk at 4.5 miles per hour (high intensity). Other activities are never high intensity, such as bowling or golf, but are still important forms of physical activity. Exercise does not need to be intense to be effective, but to lose fat it must be sustained. In the beginning you may be able to sustain exercise for only ten minutes. That is fine. Start at a point where you are comfortable and then build up your exercise tolerance from there.

There are four heart rate measurements fitness specialists use to monitor health and determine a person's appropriate heart rate during exercise.

- Resting heart rate: The number of times your heart beats per minute when at rest.
- Ambient heart rate: The number of times your heart beats per minute when you are up and moving throughout the day.
- Maximum heart rate: The number of times your heart beats per minute during maximum exercise or exertion.
- Recovery heart rate: The number of times your heart beats per minute after stopping aerobic exercise.

Calculating and Monitoring Your Heart Rate

Heart rate is expressed in number of beats per minute (bpm). You measure your heart rate by counting each beat for one minute. It is best to measure your heart rate a few times and then take the average of the measures. Resting heart rate is best measured when you first wake up in the morning, before you get out of bed. Your body performs best and is at lower risk for health problems if your resting heart rate is below 60 beats per minute. A lower resting heart rate means that your heart is not working as hard to pump the same amount of blood through your body. If your resting heart rate is 80 bpm, your heart needs to pump 20 more times per minute to move the same amount of blood as it would if your resting heart rate was 60 bpm.

Your ambient heart rate is your heart rate when you are engaged in normal daily activities. As you increase physical activity, your heart rate increases. Walking around the house increases heart rate easily to more than 90 bpm. During your daily moderate-level walk it may go up to 130 bpm, sometimes more if you are walking on hills or in the heat, or if you are fatigued. When you come back from your walk and stretch, it usually decreases below 90 bpm. As you can see, your heart rate is on a continuum. Your heart rate passes through a number of heart "zones" as your activity increases and decreases throughout the day or during your workout as you increase intensity or speed. You can monitor your progress by paying attention to your resting, ambient, and recovery heart rates. As you become fitter and your heart becomes more efficient, these measurements will decrease and your heart rate will reach its recovery rate quicker.

Your Heart Rate "Zones"

Exercise experts have determined that you get different benefits from different levels of exercise. It is best to exercise in a variety of what is called "heart rate zones" than in only one zone. Calculating your individual training zones begins by estimating your maximum heart rate. All of your exercise heart zones will be based on this number. Your maximum heart rate is the maximum number of beats your heart can beat in a minute while exercising. Your maximum heart rate:

- is genetically determined—you are born with it
- cannot be increased by training
- declines with age only in relatively sedentary individuals
- does not predict better athletic performance
- does not predict your fitness level
- varies greatly among people of the same age
- can be predicted by a mathematical formula

To *estimate* your maximum heart rate, you subtract your age from 220. It's that simple. Based on your maximum heart rate, you can calculate your individual training zones. Be aware that because you have only an estimation of your maximum heart rate, you may need to adjust your zones. Your true maximum heart rate may be higher or lower. If it is higher than what you estimated, you will not be exercising with enough intensity. If it is lower than what you estimated, you will be exercising too hard.

If you want to find out your true maximum heart rate, you must take a test either by a trained physician on a treadmill or devise your own test. Maximum heart rate tests and submaximum heart rate tests you can do safely at home are found in either of Sally Edwards's two books, *Heart Zone Training* and *Heart Rate Monitor Guide Book to Heart Zone Training* (see Appendix b). Here is the one-mile walking submaximum heart rate test found in *Heart Zone Training*.

Go to any high school or college track (most are 400 meters or 440 yards around) and walk or stride. Don't use race-walking technique with huge arm swings and hip rotations, just your normal, comfortable walking style. Walk four continuous, evenly paced and vigorous laps (1 mile). The first three laps will put you on a heart rate plateau or steady state, where you will remain for the last lap.

The last lap is the important one. Determine your average heart rate for only the last lap. Add to this average last-lap rate the number that best matches your current fitness condition:

- Add 40 bpm if you are in poor shape (you do not exercise at all or have not exercised in the past eight weeks).
- Add 50 bpm if you are in average shape (you walk a mile three times a week or you participate in any aerobic activity three times per week for twenty minutes).
- Add 60 bpm if you are in excellent shape (you exercise more than one hour a week or you walk or run at least five miles a week).

Figure 14.1. The effects of "yo-yo" dieting on muscle loss and fat gain

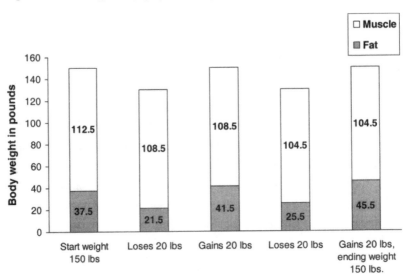

Graph design by Clayton Hibbert.

For example, a person in poor shape might have an average heart rate of 120 bpm for the last lap. Adding 40 bpm to that makes a maximum heart rate of 160 bpm. A person in average shape might record 125 bpm for the last lap, then add 50 bpm for a total of 175. A person in excellent shape would add 60 beats to her rate of 135 bpm for a maximum heart rate of 195.

There are five exercise heart zones from which you can choose. You get different benefits in each zone.

Tip for Breast Cancer Patients and Survivors

It is best to wait six months to a year following chemotherapy before performing a maximum or submaximum heart rate test. You will not hurt yourself in any way by performing a test earlier; you just may not be able to bring your heart rate up to get an accurate measurement due to muscle loss or treatment side effects. This may be frustrating. Exercising in the wellness zones (zone 1 and zone 2) will allow for gentle recovery and increase your overall endurance. As you recover and regain muscle strength, you should gradually start to exercise in the higher heart zones. Once you feel you have regained enough strength to exert yourself, try a submax or max heart rate test.

Zone 1: Healthy Heart Zone

In zone 1, your heart rate stays at about 50 to 60 percent of your maximum heart rate. Zone 1 provides low-intensity exercise for those with wellness goals or beginning an exercise program. If done for a long enough duration and frequency, exercising in this zone can reduce blood pressure, improve cholesterol levels, stabilize body fat, and improve muscle mass. For more serious athletes, this is the best zone for warm-up and cooldown.

Table 14.2. Heart Zone Chart

How to Read This Chart:

1. Heart rates are expressed in beats per minute.
2. Determine your individual maximum heart rate (see page 183) and find this number across the top row.
3. Choose your exercise intensity goals from the Exercise Zones column. Exercise intensity is expressed as a percentage of your maximum heart rate.
4. Line up your goal and your maximum heart rate to discover your heart rate workout range.

HEART ZONES
(beats per minute)

EXERCISE ZONES (% of maximum heart rate)		MAXIMUM HEART RATE														
		150	155	160	165	170	175	180	185	190	195	200	205	210	215	220
ZONE 5	100%	150	155	160	165	170	175	180	185	190	195	200	205	210	215	220
Redline	90%	135	140	144	149	153	158	162	167	171	176	180	185	189	194	198
ZONE 4	90%	135	140	144	149	153	158	162	167	171	176	180	185	189	194	198
Threshold	80%	120	124	128	132	136	140	144	148	152	156	160	164	168	172	176
ZONE 3	80%	120	124	128	132	136	140	144	148	152	156	160	164	168	172	176
Aerobic	70%	105	109	112	116	119	123	126	130	133	137	140	144	147	151	154
ZONE 2	70%	105	109	112	116	119	123	126	130	133	137	140	144	147	151	154
Temperate	60%	90	93	96	99	102	105	108	111	114	117	120	123	126	129	132
ZONE 1	60%	90	93	96	99	102	105	108	111	114	117	120	123	126	129	132
Healthy Heart	50%	75	78	80	83	85	88	90	93	95	98	100	103	105	108	110

(WELLNESS ZONES applies to Zone 2 and Zone 1)

Source: Adapted from Sally Edwards, *The Heart Rate Monitor Guide Book to Heart Zone Training* and *Heart Zone Training*. Graph design by Clayton Hibbert.

☞ Zone 2: Temperate or Fat-Burning Zone

The heart rate range for zone 2 is 60 to 70 percent of maximum heart rate. Although exercise intensity is still moderate in zone 2, fat is burned at a higher rate than in zone 1. In zone 2 you can burn high levels of fat because you can sustain this heart rate comfortably for a longer period of time. It is sometimes called the "comfort zone." For long, sustained workouts, zone 2 is the easiest to maintain because it is at a mild intensity level.

✍   Zone 3: Aerobic Zone

Zone 3 heart rate ranges from 70 to 80 percent of maximum heart rate. The aerobic zone is known best for its capacity to improve aerobic fitness. In this zone you will burn slightly more fat than in zone 1 or zone 2. The intensity has increased so that your overall fitness also increases in this zone. It is not as comfortable as the temperate zone, so you will likely not want to stay as long at this level as at the lower levels.

✍   Zone 4: Threshold Zone

This high-intensity zone maximizes fitness improvement. It is difficult to sustain this zone, in which the heart rate is 80 to 90 percent of maximum, for very long. Even short bouts of exercise in this zone, however, make immense improvements in your fitness and performance levels. We encourage women to do interval workouts in this zone. For example, in a thirty-minute fitness walk, you may walk a few hills quickly that put you in zone 4 for two minutes on each hill. (Using hills to vary workout is an example of an interval workout.)

✍   Zone 5: Redline Zone

Zone 5 ranges from 90 to 100 percent of maximal heart rate. This high-performance zone can be sustained for only a few minutes because it brings your heart rate very close to your maximum. This zone is not primarily used for burning fat, but rather is a speed zone. For athletes wanting to perform faster, this heart zone is used in very short sessions.

✍   How to Calculate Your Zones

Here are two examples of how to calculate your heart rate zones.

Joan has been exercising for a while but has set a goal to lose some fat and get more fit. She has decided to exercise primarily in zone 3, the aerobic zone, which is between 70 and 80 percent of her maximum heart rate. After doing a submaximum heart rate test, she estimates that her maximum heart rate is 180 beats per minute. She then calculates 80 percent of 180 and 70 percent of 180 to get a zone 3 range between 126 and 144 bpm.

180 x .70 (70%) = 126
180 x .80 (80%) = 144

Suzanne is currently in breast cancer treatment and wants to exercise. She is fifty-three years old. She and her doctor have decided it would be best for her to exercise below 60 percent of her maximum heart rate throughout chemotherapy. She is choosing to stay in the wellness zones, zones 1 and 2. Since she is currently in cancer treatment, she should not do a submaximum test to estimate her maximal heart rate and should instead estimate it by subtracting her age from 220.

220 – 53 = 167

Suzanne then estimates 60 percent of her maximal heart rate as:

167 x .60 (60%) = 100 bpm

If Suzanne wants to exercise no higher than 60 percent of her maximum heart rate, she needs to keep her heart rate under 100 bpm during exercise.

Heart Rate Monitors

Heart rate monitors are biofeedback devices that make tracking your heart rate simple. A heart rate monitor measures your heart rate—the number of heartbeats in a minute. A heartbeat is one contraction of your heart muscle. When you take your pulse, you are measuring your heartbeats. Heart rate monitors measure the electrical activity of the heart. A heart rate monitor has two pieces: a chest strap that is worn against the skin as close to the heart as possible, and a wrist watchlike receiver that gives you a constant reading of your heart rate.

There are a number of benefits to using a heart rate monitor.

- It is helpful not to have to stop or slow down to take a pulse rate. You get a more accurate measurement of exercise inten-

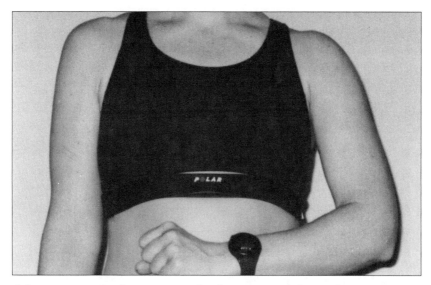

A heart-rate monitor has two parts: the chest strap and the watch.

sity with a heart rate monitor because it continually displays your heart rate on the face of the receiver unit.

• The transmitter counts your heartbeats for you and relays your rate to the wristband for easy and quick interpretation.

Figure 14.2. Type and amount of calories used in different heart rate zones, per half hour of exercise

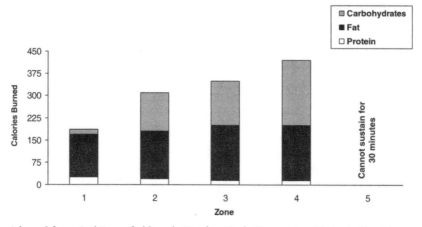

Adapted from Gail Butterfield et al., *Hershey Foods Corporation: Topics in Nutrition and Food Safety: Fueling Activity*, fall 1994, p. 6, and Sally Edwards, *Heart Rate Monitor Guide Book to Heart Zone Training*. Graph design by Clayton Hibbert.

- A heart rate monitor can act as a training partner, keeping you on pace and on track to your goal.
- A heart rate monitor is motivational and allows you to challenge yourself. An example of a healthy challenge would be to say while doing an interval workout. "Can I maintain 145 bpm for the next two minutes?" or, "Can I sustain this pace of 136 bpm all the way around the track one time?"
- Although we encourage overall goals, a heart rate monitor can help you set goals in each workout.

How Much Exercise Do You Need?

Unfortunately your doctor can't tell you, "Due to your blessed genes you need only one hour of exercise per week to stay healthy and free of disease" or, "I'm sorry, but tests show that women in your family will need an average of five hours of aerobic exercise at 70 percent of your maximum heart rate to reduce your chance of breast cancer." With our current state of knowledge, we cannot predict how much exercise each woman needs to reduce risk of breast cancer and maintain health. It is your doctor's responsibility to help you maintain and manage your good health; it is your job to find out how much exercise it takes for your body to work well and keep fit and healthy.

Keeping a Log of Your Exercise or Training Program

Maintaining a regular exercise program is best accomplished by designing a training program. A training program is different from an exercise program. In a training program you set a goal and write down a plan to reach the goal. In an exercise program you just go to the gym or walk around the lake because you enjoy staying active. Setting a goal and training to meet that goal increases your chances of sticking with your exercise plan and getting the results you want. Keeping a log helps you to plan your weekly workouts and ensures that you are maintaining regular exercise sessions. A log allows you to record your progress over time. It also provides data for any professionals who are supporting or monitoring your exercise plan, such as your doctor or fitness specialist. A tip for using a log is to write down in pencil all of the exercise sessions you are planning to do for the week. Note the exercise sessions you plan to do alone, with training buddies, and with a group or team. Then, throughout the week note in pen your workouts after they are complete. This is a good way to see if you are setting appropriate weekly goals. Analyze your log regularly and ask yourself questions such as:

- If I have not completed all of the workouts I predicted, could it be that I set my goals too high for the week?
- If I end up doing more than I plan every week, could it be that I am setting my goals too low?
- Do I do better when I am with a training buddy?

Answering these questions will help you to become proficient at planning your training program and being your own best training partner.

Sample Exercise Programs

Listed below are sample progressive exercise programs that will help you to design and write your own individualized training program. These programs are just a guide for how you can move from not exercising up to exercising about four hours a week. If you are already exercising but want more physical activity, just find where you are on the progression and start designing your exercise program from there.

Sample Program for *Any* Woman Wanting to Reduce Her Risk for Breast Cancer

Karen is as ready as she is ever going to be to begin her exercise program. She has started exercise programs many times in the past and failed to maintain them. She is motivated now since her sister's best friend was just diagnosed with breast cancer. Karen has never liked health clubs. She has decided to take up running but feels that she needs support to do this. A coworker has expressed interest in exercising at least twice a week together. Training partners are the best way to help keep you motivated and stay consistent with your program. Karen's goal is to go from her current no exercise to four hours of aerobic exercise a week.

Table 14.3 Karen's Twenty-Week Progressive Walk and Jog Program

	MONDAY	WEDNESDAY	FRIDAY	SATURDAY
Week 1	*walk* 20 MINUTES	*walk* 30 MINUTES	*walk* 20 MINUTES	
Week 2	*walk* 30	*walk* 30	*walk* 20	
Week 3	*walk* 40	*walk* 40	*walk* 30	
Week 4	*walk* 30, *jog* 5	*walk* 40	*walk* 30, *jog* 5	*walk* 30
Week 5	*walk* 45	*walk* 30, *jog* 10	*walk* 30, *jog* 5	*walk* 40
Week 6	*walk* 50	*walk* 30, *jog* 5	*walk* 50	*walk* 30, *jog* 10
Week 7	*walk* 60	*walk* 30, *jog* 10	*walk* 55	*walk* 30, *jog* 15
Week 8	*walk* 60	*walk* 30, *jog* 15	*walk* 30, *jog* 15	*walk* 60
Week 9	*walk* 30, *jog* 20	*walk* 30, *jog* 15	*walk* 60	*walk* 30, *jog* 20
Week 10	*walk* 30, *jog* 20	*walk* 60	*walk* 30, *jog* 25	*walk* 30, *jog* 25
Week 11	(out of town)	*walk* 30	*jog* 20	*jog* 30
Week 12	*walk* 60	*walk* 30, *jog* 30	*walk* 30, *jog* 30	*walk* 60
Week 13	*walk* 25, *jog* 35	*walk* 25, *jog* 35	*walk* 60	*walk* 20, *jog* 40
Week 14	*walk* 20, *jog* 40	*walk* 60	*walk* 15, *jog* 45	*walk* 20, *jog* 40
Week 15	*walk* 60	*walk* 15, *jog* 45	*walk* 15, *jog* 45	*walk* 60
Week 16	*walk* 10, *jog* 50	*walk* 15, *jog* 45	*walk* 60	*walk* 10, *jog* 50
Week 17	*walk* 10, *jog* 50	*walk* 60	*walk* 5, *jog* 55	*walk* 10, *jog* 50
Week 18	*walk* 60	*walk* 5, *jog* 55	*walk* 60	*walk* 60
Week 19	*walk* 50, *jog* 10	*jog* 60	*walk* 60	*walk* 5, *jog* 55
Week 20	*jog* 60	*walk* 60	*jog* 60	*jog* 60

Sample Exercise Program for a Woman Currently in Breast Cancer Treatment

Helen is forty-five years old and experienced early menopause as a result of her breast cancer treatment. Her only exercise has been an aerobics class twice a week. She had been doing the aerobics class for three years before she was diagnosed but hasn't been to class for three months since starting treatment. Helen is experiencing an average amount of fatigue due to her mastectomy, chemotherapy, and radiation treatments. She has most of her shoulder range of motion back after her breast surgery. She works full-time and takes care of her two teenage sons.

Helen begins by doing a stretching program that will improve her upper body range of motion but includes trunk and lower body stretching too. She does her stretching program for forty-five minutes twice a week. She does this at the gym where she used to take her aerobics class. She starts her aerobic program by riding the stationary bike for ten minutes. The bike has a built in heart rate monitor so she can constantly monitor her heart rate and keep it below the recommended 65 percent max. Since she is forty-five years old, her estimated maximum heart rate is 175. Sixty-five percent of that is 114, so she needs to keep her heart rate below 114 when she exercises. Slowly she builds her bike workout up to ten minutes four times per week over the next month.

Helen has added another stretch workout. She then begins riding the bike a little longer, increasing the duration by two to four minutes every other time. She can ride up to twenty minutes now but not more because of fatigue. She discovered if she rides longer she is more tired the next day. Helen is now riding the bike twenty minutes four times per week. She started by first increasing frequency and increased the duration only after she had success with no increased fatigue. Next she increased her duration until she found a comfortable amount of exercise. She will keep the intensity at 65 percent of her maximum heart rate for two to four weeks. Even on a good day, when she is experiencing minimal treatment side effects, if she rides too fast and gets her heart rate too high she finds she needs to sleep longer the next day and take more than one nap.

Table 14.4. Helen's Twelve-Week Progressive Indoor Bike Program

	MONDAY	WEDNESDAY	FRIDAY	SATURDAY
Week 1	10 minutes	10 minutes		
Week 2	10 minutes	10 minutes		
Week 3	10 minutes	10 minutes	10 minutes	
Week 4	10 minutes	10 minutes	10 minutes	10 minutes
Week 5*				

*At week 5 Helen's blood cell counts were down from the chemotherapy, and she had only enough energy to do her stretching program at home.

	MONDAY	WEDNESDAY	FRIDAY	SATURDAY
Week 6	10 minutes	10 minutes	10 minutes	
Week 7	10 minutes	10 minutes	10 minutes	10 minutes
Week 8	12 minutes	10 minutes	12 minutes	10 minutes
Week 9	12 minutes	14 minutes	12 minutes	14 minutes
Week 10	17 minutes	14 minutes	17 minutes	14 minutes
Week 11	17 minutes	20 minutes	17 minutes	20 minutes
Week 12	20 minutes	20 minutes	20 minutes	20 minutes

Sample Exercise Program for a Woman Recently Recovering from Breast Cancer Treatment

It has been eight weeks since Helen's last radiation treatment. Helen is experiencing an expected amount of physical and emotional fatigue for this stage. She is most interested in weight loss now and wants to lose the fifteen pounds she put on over the last year of treatment. She is still exercising on the indoor bike four times a week for twenty minutes. Her exercise goal is to progress to a training plan for fat loss that ultimately includes three exercise sessions a week with at least of two them being forty-five minutes of aerobic exercise.

Table 14.5. Helen's Twelve-Week Progressive Exercise Program

	MONDAY	WEDNESDAY	FRIDAY
Week 1	*bike* 20 MINUTES, *walk* 5 MINUTES	*bike* 20 MINUTES	*bike* 20 MINUTES, *walk* 20 MINUTES
Week 2	*bike* 20, *walk* 5	*bike* 20, *walk* 5	*bike* 20, *walk* 20
Week 3	*bike* 20, *walk* 10	*bike* 20, *walk* 10, *bike* 20	*walk* 20
Week 4	*bike* 20, *walk* 10	*bike* 20, *walk* 10, *bike* 20	*walk* 25
Week 5	*bike* 20, *walk* 10	*bike* 20, *walk* 10, *bike* 20	*walk* 25
Week 6	*bike* 20, *walk* 10	*bike* 20, *walk* 10, *bike* 20	*walk* 30
Week 7	*bike* 20, *walk* 15	*bike* 20, *walk* 10, *bike* 20	*walk* 30
Week 8	*bike* 20, *walk* 15	*bike* 20, *walk* 15, *bike* 20	*walk* 30
Week 9	*bike* 20, *walk* 15	*bike* 20, *walk* 15, *bike* 20	*walk* 30
Week 10	*bike* 20. *walk* 15	*bike* 20, *walk* 15, *bike* 20	*walk* 35
Week 11	*bike* 20, *walk* 15	*bike* 20, *walk* 15, *bike* 20	*walk* 40
Week 12	*bike* 20, *walk* 15	*bike* 20, *walk* 15, *bike* 20	*walk* 45

Increasing Your Exercise Intensity

Once your exercise frequency and duration have met your goals, the next step is to add intensity. Intensity can be measured either by your heart rate range or training zone. Think about what you want from your exercise plan and match your frequency, duration, and intensity to your goal.

Goal: Losing Fat

Plan: Sustained aerobic exercise for thirty to sixty minutes four to five times per week:

- One workout each week of low intensity for longer duration
- One workout of higher intensity for a shorter duration
- Two to three workouts of moderate intensity and longer durations

For example:

Monday	Zone 1	60 minutes
Tuesday	Zone 3	30 minutes
Thursday	Zone 2	45 minutes
Friday	Zone 2	60 minutes
Sunday	Zone 2	45 minutes

Goal: Maintaining Body Weight and Increasing Fitness

This is for the woman who is happy with her body weight and fat, and is interested in a leaner-looking body and improving her exercise performance.

Plan: Sustained aerobic exercise for forty-five minutes five times per week:

- Two workouts at an aerobic endurance pace
- One strength workout using two zones
- One longer and lower-intensity workout
- One shorter and faster workout

For example:

Monday	Zone 2	60 minutes
Tuesday	Zone 3 and zone 4	45 minutes
Wednesday	Zone 3	45 minutes

| Friday | Zone 3 and zone 4 | 30 minutes |
| Sunday | Zone 3 | 45 minutes |

Goal: Maintaining Body Size, Shape, and Fitness
This is for the woman who has little time to think about her exercise program, is happy with her body weight and exercise capacity, and is interested in simply maintaining.
Plan: Sustained aerobic exercise for at least forty-five minutes five times per week:

- Five comfortable, endurance-pace workouts per week

For example:

Monday	Zone 2	45 minutes
Tuesday	Zone 2	45 minutes
Wednesday	Zone 1	60 minutes
Thursday	Zone 2	45 minutes
Saturday	Zone 1	60 minutes

Summary

- The research data give us limited information on exactly what women need to do to reduce their risk of breast cancer, but they point to the importance of vigorous exercise in teen and adult years and to prevention of excess fat gain with aging.
- At least some of your exercise should be aerobic, cause sweating, result in a heart rate that is consistent with your goals, and be done daily or almost every day.
- Breast cancer patients should stay below 65 percent of maximum estimated heart rate while they are undergoing treatment. They should not measure their maximum heart rate at this time but should use the estimated value.
- Exercise has three main components: frequency, duration, and intensity.
- You need to decide what your goals are with exercise before

you can design an exercise or training program that will work for you.

- Heart zone training is an excellent method to help you monitor your exercise intensity.
- A heart rate monitor is a simple way for you to know your heart rate at all times during exercise and can help you to stay in the zone that fits your particular goals.

15

Setting Exercise Goals for Each Stage of Your Life

Many women have asked us exactly what exercises they should do to reduce risk of breast cancer. The truth is that no one particular exercise is likely to be the answer. Rather, the important thing is to follow an individual exercise and diet plan that will help you reach goals associated with optimal breast health—reduced chance of breast cells becoming cancerous and reduced stimulation of existing cancer cells. The benefits of following such a plan also include positive effects on other aspects of your health, including reduced risk of obesity, heart disease, diabetes, hypertension, colon cancer, and osteoarthritis, and perhaps increased immune function and improved intellectual and emotional well-being. In this chapter we describe the results you should aim for, depending on your age and whether you have gone through menopause. For women at each of four life stages corresponding to ages, we give guidance on goals for exercise. The four groups are (1) girls and teens; (2) young and premenopausal women: (3) pregnant women or women planning to get pregnant; and (4) women going through or past menopause. We talk about goals for maintaining a healthy weight and level of fitness throughout life.

In Chapter 6, we told you about the mechanisms through which exercise might reduce risk of new or recurrent breast cancer. The amount of exercise needed may vary by mechanism; thus we recommend that each woman maximize her activity level according to her own ability and time constraints. In general, greater-intensity exercise gives more "bang for the buck"—it results in greater energy expenditure and better control of body fat stores. The old adage of doing twenty minutes of aerobic activity three times per week is not likely to be enough to control fat stores and reduce hormone levels to a degree that would provide protection against breast cancer. For most women, thirty to sixty minutes per day of aerobic activity are needed, combined with a judicious diet. To aid with control of body fat and to improve strength, we also recommend a program of muscle strengthening.

You can test your body fat using a machine that measures bioelectric impedance. Many health clubs have a bioelectric impedance machine. Or you can purchase a handheld one yourself for about $100. A bioelectric impedance test measures two different "body components": your total body mass and your fat-free mass. The fat-free mass includes muscle, cells, and other body structures that are not fat. The machine then calculates the percent of your body that is made of fat. These measures are made by passing a very weak electrical current through your body, similar to the way an electrocardiogram works. It is completely safe and gives you a good idea of how much body fat you have in proportion to the rest of your body. Women tend to have higher percentages of body fat than men, and older persons have higher percentages of body fat than younger persons. Many women who do not exercise, and who gain fat mass through the years, can have 50 percent or more of their bodies consisting of fat! We recommend that you keep your body fat to between 22 to 28 percent or less throughout your life.

Girls and Teens

For girls and young teens who have not yet begun to menstruate, the goal for breast protection is to delay the age at onset of menstrual periods while at the same time increasing muscle mass to help protect bones. The best way to do this is to avoid excess gain of fat and to maximize physical activity, usually from sports and recreational exercise. Weight-bearing sports help to develop strong bones. Many sports include high-intensity exercise, or long hours of moderate-intensity exercise, which can reduce the chance of excess fat storage. High-intensity sports are those in which the participant sweats and has a significant increase in heart rate while engaged in the activity. A measure that is used to deter-

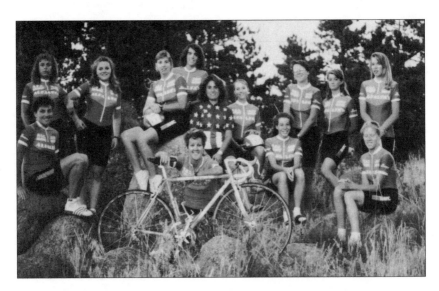

Cycling is a great form of exercise for young women. Karen Hornbostel (center, holding the bike) and her cycling team. Photo: Karen Hornbostel.

mine the intensity of an exercise or sport is the "met level," which is the metabolic rate for a specific activity divided by the resting metabolic rate. The metabolic rate sitting quietly at rest is arbitrarily defined as 1.0. An activity that has a met level of 2 requires twice the amount of energy as sitting quietly at rest. In Appendix A we show the met level for various sports and activities. Sports and activities with a met level greater than 6.0 are considered high intensity; these include basketball, hockey, track, and competitive swimming. Girls who participate in these types of sports typically have low levels of body fat and do not start to menstruate until they are thirteen years old or later. Parents have to be very careful, however, about the messages they give to their sports-involved daughters about weight control. Often, girls participating in competitive sports are urged by coaches to lose weight. Girls can internalize this urging to the extent that they reduce weight to unhealthy levels. This can result in excessively low body weights, very low estrogen levels, osteoporosis, and fractures. The best advice for parents who want to promote optimal breast health for their daughters is to encourage participation in sports and to provide nutritious foods at home with minimal amounts of calorie-laden junk foods available. In cases where a girl is clearly obese or overweight, a weight-loss program should be undertaken under the guidance of a pediatrician or family physician.

Young and Premenopausal Women

For young women and for women who have not yet gone through menopause, the main goal is to prevent lifetime accumulation of fat and to maintain muscle and bone mass. For most women, yearly accumulation of fat results in a weight gain of two to three pounds per year or more after the twenties. (This doesn't sound like very much, but after ten years it amounts to twenty to thirty pounds.) Many women who are physically active in their teen years slow down as they take on sedentary jobs and start their families. Most occupations in the United States today can be considered sedentary, and the trend is to increase the sedentary aspects of most jobs while increasing availability and use of labor-saving technology. We tend to expend less energy getting to work, as so many of us commute by automobile. At work, we use elevators rather than stairs, and we communicate via E-mail rather than walking to a colleague's office. At home, women tend to spend more time driving the kids to their activities and less time with physically demanding housework than in previous decades. If your dietary calorie intake remains the same as it was in your teen years, but your level of physical activity decreases, the result will be a steady gain in body fat stores that show up on the scale as increased weight.

A secondary goal for premenopausal women is to reduce the number of menstrual cycles that are accompanied by ovulation (release of an egg). By reducing the number of cycles with ovulation, levels of estrogen and progesterone are decreased, thus decreasing the stimulation of breast cells. Since you probably have no idea whether you ovulated in a particular month, the goal is to exercise at a high enough level to produce an effect on ovulation. You may even notice that the length of time between your cycles increases. Or you may notice that you have less bleeding or fewer days of bleeding. You may not notice any change in your cycle pattern, or you may notice some irregular bleeding, or bleeding between periods. If you experience a change in menstrual habits, you should check with your gynecologist or family doctor, but realize that a change in menstrual pattern may be a sign that your increase in exercise is having an effect on your body's hormone patterns.

Women Planning to Become Pregnant

If you are actively trying to get pregnant you should talk with your doctor before increasing your level of aerobic physical activity, since you do not want to reduce your chances of ovulating and getting pregnant.

Pregnant Women

If your doctor or midwife says that exercise is okay for you during your pregnancy, you can continue to do many of your prepregnancy activities. There are some things you should keep in mind, however. You are carrying a baby in your abdominal area. While your body provides an excellent shield for it, there is not a guaranteed protection. Activities or sports that increase risk for trauma put your baby at considerable risk. Activities that are probably too risky for a pregnant women include anything with high speed or that is done at great heights. You may have been a first-class rock climber before you became pregnant. However, the hormonal changes and tendency to pool blood in your lower extremities may make you dizzy or woozy at times. If that happens while you are climbing, you would be at risk for falling and injury. Repetitive stress, such as from jogging, can put

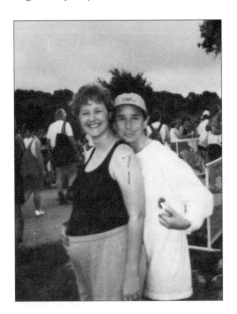

Staying active and exercising during pregnancy help you maintain your health and manage postnatal weight gain.

excessive strain on your uterine ligaments. It is likely better to switch to brisk walking by your second trimester. You should also avoid an increase in core temperature (that might happen with exercise in extreme heat), extreme exhaustion, or dehydration. Scuba diving and mountain climbing can pose risk to the baby or you because of low oxygen availability. Don't use your heart rate to gauge your intensity—better to use your perceived level of exertion. If you can talk normally while doing the activity, then the intensity level is probably fine.

Some good activities for pregnant women are brisk and moderate walking, bicycling (through the second trimester), golf, cross-country skiing (through second trimester), swimming (up until the end of your eighth month), low-impact aerobics, and yoga (some positions are not safe for pregnant women—check with your doctor or midwife). Stretching exercises and lower-back stretches can help with the aches and pains of pregnancy and can aid in the baby's delivery.

Gynecologists warn, however, that women with any of the following conditions should not exercise during pregnancy: congestive heart failure, certain types of valvular heart disease, severe hypertension, uterine bleeding, premature rupture of membranes, or incompetent cervix.

Women Going Through Menopause and Postmenopausal Women

During and after menopause, you should aim to reduce body fat stores so that your body fat is at 28 percent or less. At the same time you should do regular muscle-building exercises to maintain muscle mass. Your optimal aerobic exercise should be weight bearing to help strengthen bones.

The best research studies have shown that increasing exercise is the best way that women can keep their body fat low, and the best way to lose body fat permanently once they have accumulated too much. Many researchers believe that the one thing that best accounts for the increasing prevalence of overweight and obesity in our society is the decrease in energy requirements of our most basic daily activities. Since most Americans' daily activities take less energy than did those of their parents or grandparents, they need fewer food calories to supply that energy. While our energy expenditure has decreased, however, our food intake

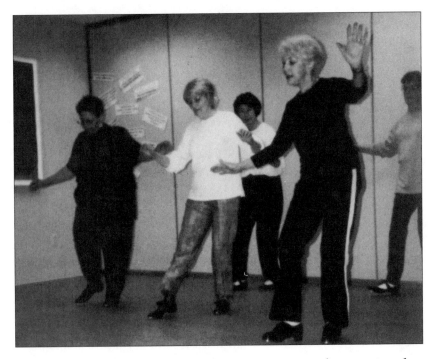

Tap dancing is fun aerobic exercise women can maintain as they move into the menopausal years. Photo: Lisa Talbott.

has not. The result is the accumulation of body fat. Look at the following table to see some examples of differences in energy required for various daily activities in women at different times in this century.

Table 15-1. Estimated Calories Burned per Hour by Women in Various Activities

ACTIVITY/NUMBER OF CALORIES BURNED					
	1920s		1950s		2000s
Laundry	Scrubbing boards, hang dry	230*	Washing machine, hang dry	140	Automatic washer and dryer 120
Grocery shopping	Walk to store 1 mile, shop 30 minutes	250	Drive to store, shop 30 minutes	125	Internet grocery shopping 0
Cleaning	Beat rugs, scrub floors	325	Vacuum cleaner	150	Hire cleaning service 0

ACTIVITY/NUMBER OF CALORIES BURNED

	1920s		1950s		2000s	
Cooking	Tend coal or wood stove, bake bread	200	Most meals prepared from scratch, some electric appliances	150	Home-delivered meals	50
Care for children	Children at home	200	Children at home	200	Full-time daycare	0
Recreation	Social events requiring cooking; radio; reading	125	Dancing, ballroom	175	Television/ VCR with remote control	75

*Calories burned per hour for a woman weighing about 130 pounds.

There are several ways that you can break this cycle. You can take in fewer calories and match your usual energy expenditure. This will reduce weight gain, though you will need to be vigilant in making sure that as you get older, you reduce your food intake even further since your metabolism likely slows with aging. Reducing food calories below daily energy requirements can result in weight loss if you want to lose the extra fat pounds you have gained over time. There are several problems with approaching weight loss through calorie reduction alone, however.

When you restrict calories below your metabolic and energy needs, you lose muscle bulk and strength along with fat mass. Losing muscle has several negative consequences. First, you feel weaker since your muscles are less powerful. You may notice that you have less strength to do some of your usual activities, such as carrying groceries or going up stairs. Second, muscles use up energy at a much faster rate than do other body tissues. So if your muscles get smaller, you burn off fewer fat calories during your usual daily activities. The result is that when you regain the weight, as most dieters eventually do, it will be in the form of more body fat.

If you diet off and on over the years, that is, if you are what we call a "yo-yo" dieter, you can end up having a very large percent of your body made up of fat tissue. With small muscles resulting from losing muscles during periods of starvation, you are carrying around a great deal of non-functioning weight in the form of fat.

After menopause, you may find that you gain fat around the middle part of your body whereas when you were younger you gained it mainly in your hips and thighs. This is because estrogens tend to promote fat deposits in the hips and thighs, producing a pear-like body shape. Male hormones like testosterone, on the other hand, promote fat deposits around the waist and abdomen, producing an apple-like body shape. As you get older, your ratio of estrogen to testosterone decreases, which causes you to accumulate more abdominal fat. The fat that is deposited in the abdominal and waist areas, especially that which is deposited around the internal organs, is the most dangerous type of fat to have in excess. We know that people who have extra fat in the abdominal area are at increased risk of having high cholesterol and high insulin levels. High levels of these substances can lead to diabetes, heart disease, and other illnesses. High insulin levels may also increase the risk of developing breast cancer, perhaps by stimulating the growth of cancer cells. There is some evidence that fat in the abdominal area is the most dangerous for increasing risk of breast cancer after menopause, as we described in Chapter 2.

The good news is that aerobic exercise is especially effective at combating fat deposits in the waist and abdominal areas. Furthermore, exercise is an excellent way to reduce the amount of fat stored around internal organs. In several studies around the world, when overweight or obese individuals were assigned by chance to an aerobic exercise program (versus no exercise or stretching only), they lost significant amounts of fat and the fat was preferentially lost in the abdominal area. Indeed, people with diabetes who exercise to lose weight may have to lose only three to four pounds of this intraabdominal fat in order to experience improvements in their glucose levels and requirements for medication. We don't know if this small amount of fat loss translates into improvements in breast cancer risk. For now, we advise women that more is probably better. They should aim for the most exercise they can realistically fit into their lifestyles, while following a judicious diet to maintain body fat at 28 percent or less.

We want to point out here that abdominal "spot" exercises such as crunches and sit-ups do not reduce fat stores in the abdominal areas. They strengthen the abdominal muscles, resulting in a slimmer abdomen appearance. You'll need to follow a regular aerobic exercise program to reduce fat in the abdomen and keep it off on a long-term basis. See Chapter 19 for more information on abdominal exercise.

The goal, then, for postmenopausal women is to reduce excess body fat, especially in the abdominal and waist areas. For most women, this requires a regular aerobic exercise program. You will likely get the best results and benefits if you include a weight-training program to increase muscle bulk and limit caloric intake to what your body needs to maintain a steady metabolic state (that is, to avoid gain of body fat). Controlling caloric intakes does not mean dieting. Instead, it means eating a varied and balanced diet that includes all of the essential nutrients (protein, carbohydrates, fiber, fats, vitamins, and minerals) with a minimum of low-nutrition junk foods such as sweets and packaged snack foods. In Chapters 18 to 20 we provide some sample aerobic and weight-training plans. In Chapter 7 we gave you nutrition guidelines. We provided examples of different ways that you might choose to meet your goals depending on your age. Keep in mind that each woman is different—what works for your friend or even your sister may not work for you. You can use our guidelines and examples and modify them to apply to your own body and lifestyle.

All Women

For women of all ages, exercise can benefit the immune system. While little is known about how the immune system might affect risk of cancer, we do know that some people with impaired immune systems are at increased risk of developing certain types of cancer. In the laboratory setting, immune cells fight breast cancer cells. So we can make a leap of faith that since exercise can promote a healthy immune system, and since some parts of the immune system may fight cancer cells, then it makes sense that exercise could reduce breast cancer risk by enhancing the immune system. (Chapter 6 described exercise and the immune system.) For women of all ages, the goal for enhancing the immune system through exercise is to exercise at a moderate or higher intensity level but not to overtrain. Overtraining is not a problem for the vast majority of women. If you are an athlete, or if you are exercising more than two hours every day, you should talk with a sports medicine physician about how you can recognize if you are overtraining to the point of causing or increasing risk for illness. For the rest of us, the amount of activity that we do in sports, exercise, or other daily activities should not cause any harm to the immune system. If you have a disorder or disease of your immune system, see your physician before increasing your current level of activity. Even people with severe immune diseases, such as AIDS, however, may gain health benefits through an exercise program.

Summary

- In general, more exercise is better. Plan to do the maximum that fits in your own lifestyle.
- Most women need to do aerobic exercise for thirty to sixty minutes per day to control body fat.
- In girls and teens, the goal is to delay the age at which periods start. Parents and coaches must monitor girls' weight, activity, and diet for early signs of excessively low weight, which can have severe and permanent deleterious effects.
- In young and premenopausal women, the goal is to reduce the number of menstrual cycles that include ovulation and to lengthen the time between menstrual periods.
- In women who are going through or have gone through menopause, the goal is to reduce excessive body fat levels. If body fat is currently at an acceptable level, the goal is to prevent gain in body fat and to maintain or increase muscle size. Body fat around the waist and abdomen may be the most important to control.
- For women of all ages, the goal is to prevent the gain of body fat over the lifespan.
- The best ways to control body fat over the long term are with aerobic and weight-training exercise.

16

Using Goals to Stay Motivated

It's not difficult to start an exercise program. The first week of January is usually a very busy time for gyms and fitness clubs, as people try to make good on their New Year's resolutions. The challenge comes with keeping up the exercise program and making it a routine part and high priority of your life. This chapter gives you tips and strategies for getting motivated to keep at your exercise program. The first and most important step is to define your goals—what you want to get out of exercise. Defining your goals helps you to monitor what you do and helps you keep on track with accomplishing your goals.

Setting Goals

If you're a typical, busy woman, you go about your daily life without thinking about what parts of your daily routine include physical activity. You may have trouble identifying what behaviors you need to change to increase your physical activity. Setting goals will help you to identify what you need to do.

Many women try to make several changes at one time without having appropriate goals in place. For example, Jane decides to start a workout program that will include forty-five minutes of fast walking or jogging each day plus weight training with hand weights three days per week. On day 1 she jogs for forty-five minutes, and that goes pretty well. On day 2

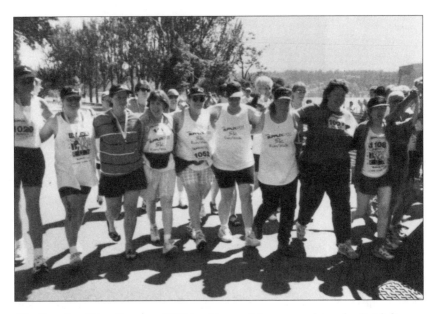

The Danskin Team Survivor Walking Team celebrates reaching the finish line and their goal. Photo: Lisa Talbott.

she jogs again for forty-five minutes and also lifts weights for thirty minutes. On day 3 she repeats the day 2 workout. On day 4 she has so much pain in her muscles and tendons that she can barely get out of bed. So she stops doing anything for three days. On day 7 she starts to jog again, then remembers the pain she had earlier in the week and stops, saying, "Oh, what's the use? I'll never be fit." So she heads home to her refrigerator and attacks a quart of ice cream instead. Jane's problem was that she tried to take on too much at once. It was too much for her body, her lifestyle, and her emotions.

It is best to select one thing to change, then write it down. After you are comfortable with your initial changes, and your body has had time to strengthen and adapt, add more activity. Set your goals close to your current level of activity. Goals should be specific, realistic, and flexible. Here are some examples of appropriate goals for women with different levels of current activity:

- Women who have never exercised and would like to start
  Goal: To start a regular walking program

- Women who have exercised in the past but are not exercising now

  Goal: To get back to taking aerobics three times a week
- Women who are exercising now but would like to do more exercise

  Goal: To increase running from three times per week to five times per week
- Women who are happy with their exercise program but need ongoing motivation

  Goal: To run a marathon

✐ Be Specific and Write It Down

Think about the activity change that you are going to make and write down exactly what you plan to do. For example, if you want to add ten minutes of walking, think about when and where you'll walk and what will be your alternative (for example, if it is raining). Write this down explicitly. For example, "At my lunch break before I eat lunch, I plan go outside, and walk for four blocks away from my office then turn around and come back." This goal is more measurable than one that says, "I want to start a walking program." Being specific about defining your goals will help you to reach them.

✐ Be Flexible

Don't set a goal that requires you to be perfect. For example, "I'll walk for ten minutes every day." "Every day" implies that you need to meet your goal all of the time, even if you are sick or have competing demands in your day. This type of goal often sets you up for failure and can produce negative feelings about the activity and guilt for taking time for yourself to exercise. Instead, you should build allowances into your goals for illness and other things going on in your life. If you are sick, your body needs to rest. If your boss needs that report, you might try to walk for ten minutes before or after work.

✍ Be Realistic

Write down the steps that you need to reach your goal. This is your action plan. Be sure to consider any steps you need to take to deal with the people and situations that might influence your activity program. Make sure that you are aware of your own feelings about exercising. Take a minute to look at your goal. Is it realistic? One way to review your goal is to pretend that a friend has shown you this same goal and is asking for your advice about it. She has the same set of challenges that you have. Knowing all of this, would you set the same goal for her? If your answer is no, then maybe you need to rethink your own goal.

After you write down your goal, make a specific action plan about how you will achieve the goal, then review them together. Make sure that your goal is specific enough so that you can measure your success. Plan to measure your progress at the same time each week. If you reach your first goal, decide what you need to do to maintain the activity changes you make that week. If you didn't succeed at your goal for that week, review what went wrong and decide what you need to do to be successful. Or review the goal to see if it was unrealistic. Below are examples of unrealistic and realistic exercise goals.

- You currently do not have an exercise program. You think that swimming would be a good activity for you because you enjoyed swimming as a child. *Unrealistic goal:* This week I will swim every day for forty-five minutes. *Realistic goal:* This week I will buy a bathing suit, visit health clubs and Y's that have free swims and offer lessons, and have two fifteen-minute lessons.
- You had a baby six months ago and feel that it's time to get back in shape. Up until your third month of pregnancy, you ran about fifteen miles per week. *Unrealistic goal:* I will pick up were I left off and run fifteen miles this week. *Realistic goal:* This week I will buy a running stroller for the baby. I will go for a twenty-minute brisk walk twice this week.
- Your grandchildren are getting harder to lift (even accounting for their normal growth). You want to be able to lift the toddler when you baby-sit. You had a mastectomy two years ago,

you have chronic swelling in your arm, and you don't have much strength at all in that arm. *Unrealistic goal:* I will use my husband's eight-pound weights and lift them every day. *Realistic goal:* This week I will start doing the Dyna-Band exercises the physical therapist taught me when I had surgery. I will ask her to help me develop a program of strength training that is safe.

- You have two children, one in middle school. You work mornings, then are home in the afternoon to take your son Johnny to his activities. Three afternoons a week he has soccer practice for one hour. *Unrealistic goal:* This week each day after I drop Johnny off, I will rush to the gym and work on the Stairmaster for thirty-five minutes, cool down, then rush to pick him up. *Realistic goal:* This week on three days while Johnny plays soccer, I will walk around the field for fifteen minutes. I will invite some of the other moms to join me.

Monitoring and Recording Your Progress

A key element for adopting and maintaining an exercise program is to keep a log of what you do. Keeping a log has several benefits.

- You can see your progress over time.
- By knowing that you are writing it down, you are more likely to do the exercise and to do it at a higher intensity, like having a running competition with yourself.
- If you have someone watching what you are doing, such as a friend or trainer, you can show off your progress and get advice for improvement.
- Keeping a log where you see it—like on the fridge—is a good reminder to do your exercise.
- You can log all parts of your routine, so you are more likely to remember to stretch and cool down, both of which are extremely important parts of exercise.
- If you are not getting the results you hoped for, logging your workouts helps you trouble-shoot your program.

Identify How You Feel About Exercise

Be aware of how you feel about exercise. Many women were taught when they were young that girls should not exert themselves in sports or other activities. Many women were just not encouraged to become athletic. Their mothers were not athletic or sports oriented, so they did not have role models on which to pattern fitness and sports. Some women have "all or none" thinking—they set perfectionist goals for themselves and if they do not meet those goals every day, they feel they have failed and just stop exercising altogether. If they cannot do the whole program they've set out for themselves, they feel they have failed and might as well stop trying. You can overcome these internal barriers to exercise and fitness. We have worked with many women who have been sedentary for forty or fifty years or more and who have successfully adopted an exercise program, increased their cardiovascular fitness, increased their muscle bulk, and lost significant amounts of body fat. You certainly are not a failure if you miss a few days of exercise as long as you do not lose sight of your goal.

Identify What Contributes to Your Success (or Lack of Success)

Identify things that can influence your success and motivate you. This could be a person such as a walking partner or an instructor at the gym you go to. Even new exercise clothes can keep women interested in their exercise program. To stay motivated it is important to continuously find things to make your feel good about your exercise program and make sure you keep these influences. You must also pay attention to what "demotivates" or contributes to your lack of success. For example, if you come home from work dragging from exhaustion, you may not feel that you have the energy to exercise, so you don't even try. More likely, you might start snacking as soon as you get home and continue all the way to bedtime. Try instead to have a small snack when you get home, such as fruit or some crackers. Then grab a bottle of water and go outside for a short walk. Paying attention to what gets in the way of your exercise and making an effort to remove these influences from your life will help your success.

Getting Help from Family, Friends, and Coworkers

The people around you may influence your immediate desire to exercise. Friends and family can help you achieve your goals, or they can make them more difficult to achieve. They may not want you to overexert yourself. Or they may want you to stay home and watch TV with them. Many people also celebrate holidays and vacations in sedentary activities. We will talk about ways that you can increase your energy output in all of these situations.

If your sister is a runner, and you can see how lean and fit she keeps from doing all of that high-energy exercise, it may help to motivate you. If your friends follow exercise programs, it can help you decide what you want to do and can motivate you. If you are surrounded by exercisers, use their experience to help you. You might accompany them as they do their activities, to see what it involves and if it looks like something you'd enjoy. You could bike along while your sister runs to watch her as she does her routine. If your girlfriend takes an aerobics class, go along with her to watch a session. You can also find out from them what motivates them to keep up with a fitness routine. Furthermore, their experience with avoiding injuries will help you to keep exercising pain free!

If you see your friends sitting in the break room as you are going out of the office to walk, do you really want to join them rather than walk? Or does seeing them make you feel better about the fact that you are improving your health and appearance by becoming more active? Be aware of the things that influence your desire to exercise. Make them work for you rather than against you. For example, when you see your colleagues head off to the lunchroom, ask if any of them would like to join you for a ten-minute walk, then have lunch together when you return.

When you go on a vacation, do you spend all of your time riding in the car seeing the sights? Your body may be so tired from all of that sitting that just getting out of the car at roadside viewpoints to take a picture may seem exhausting. Instead, you might try a destination vacation, where you stay in a resort or cabin and do some activities every day that take some energy, such as walking, hiking, canoeing, or biking. Many resorts have such activities readily available. If you are not used to these activities, you might want to take advantage of guided trips such as nature walks offered in some national parks. By encouraging your family to become more active with you, it will help you in your fitness goals, and it will also benefit their health!

On the other hand, if your husband is a dedicated couch potato and wants you to keep him company, it can add to the challenges facing you as you increase exercise in your life. Once you know how important your exercise program is to you, stand up for your decision to exercise. You need to be able to deal with your family and friends in an assertive way. Being assertive does not mean being selfish. You can be assertive and still be sensitive to your family members' and friends' feelings. Here are some tips for being assertive with someone who is challenging your decision to exercise.

- Don't raise your voice or whine. Use a relaxed, pleasant tone.
- Make direct eye contact. This lets them know that you mean business.
- Be clear in what you say to them. Say, "I am going to go out for my walk now," rather than, "Well, I was really hoping to go out for a walk now, but if you don't think I should I guess I could do it later."
- Invite the challenger to go along with you. If that person wanted to talk to you, say that you'd be happy to walk and talk. If one of the kids wants your attention, take him out with you or let her do the aerobics tape with you.
- Make a plan: I am going to go exercise now, but can we have dinner together when I get back?

Problem Solving

You can use problem solving as a step-by-step approach to defining and solving challenges in your exercise program. It is a method for thinking through a situation and reminding yourself of your choices about exercising. The first step in problem solving is identifying what is challenging you. For example, Sarah wants to start a fitness program. She works as a programmer for a computer software support company. Although her official hours are 8:30 to 5:00, her group frequently has projects coming up against tight deadlines, and she has to work up to eighty hours per week to make the deadlines. She is single and does not have children. There are several things in this situation that could be challenging for Sarah.

- She feels that if she starts on an exercise routine, she'll have to give it up when her group faces its next crunch time.
- She feels that she does not get enough sleep as it is during the crunch times and does not want to add another "chore" to her impossibly busy life.
- She is afraid that if she goes to exercise, or if she does not join in all of the last-minute crunch work, her boss and colleagues won't think she is dedicated enough. It could affect her promotion possibilities.
- She may be experiencing muscle pain and stiffness from long hours sitting in front of the computer. These long hours sitting may be making her more fatigued with less energy to start an exercise program.

We can use Sarah's situation to problem solve. First, determine what might be Sarah's main challenge. Sarah decides that setting priorities is the biggest problem for her. She has put the demands of her job ahead of her physical and emotional needs. Second, think about what Sarah wants to do about the problem. Sarah wants to fit exercise into her daily life, while still being able to perform well at her job. Third, think of a solution. She needs to find ways to fit exercise into her schedule. A flexible program will be key for her. Some possible solutions for her are:

- Start using the stairs at work, avoiding the elevator.
- If the parking lot is in a safe area, park at the farthest end of the lot so that she has to walk farther to get to and from the building each day.
- Do an activity that can be done in short bursts at odd hours, such as using a stationary bicycle at home.
- Take exercise breaks at work: Get up from the computer, stretch, go outside and walk around the building few times. In bad weather, walk inside the building and up and down stairs. Work up to running the stairs.
- Ask for a height-adjustable workstation, so that she can cut

down on her hours sitting. (Standing uses more energy than
sitting and is easier on the back and legs than sitting.)

- Bring weights or Dyna-Bands to work and do them while
  thinking through an algorithm or problem.

Next, think about what might happen if Sarah tries her solutions.
She needs to think about what could happen to derail any of her solutions. Some things that might go wrong:

- On day 1 she walks up all the way to her office on the seventh
  floor. She's sweating and is embarrassed when a couple of
  coworkers make a remark about it.
- She decides that she doesn't feel safe walking around the outside of her building.
- Her boss refuses to authorize the adjustable workstation.

Sarah needs to think through the pluses and minuses of each of her solutions and decide which ones will work for her. Then she needs to put her
solutions into action. After she has tried one solution, Sarah needs to
think about how it worked for her. If she is not happy with the result she
may need to try another solution.

You can use these skills to think through your own challenges to
exercise. You know that you have challenges to exercising. We all do;
even the greatest athletes face challenges in performing to their peak.

Use Positive Self-Talk and Avoid Negative Self-Talk

The ways that you think about yourself and your surroundings have profound effects on the decisions you make about your actions. Picture
yourself having had a very bad day. Your boss had you running around all
morning with a very important project that had to be finished by noon,
you have to leave work early because you couldn't find anyone to drive
your son to football practice, and your mom called you to take her to the
doctor. It's now 6:00 P.M., the time when you usually put on an aerobics
videotape in the family room and work out for a half hour. You're exhaust-

ed, however, and just want to collapse on the couch with some tea and chocolate. Let's look at some examples of positive and negative thoughts you might have about your day.

Positive thoughts:

- I feel tired, so I'll just do a low-impact program tonight.
- Since I'm tired I'll go to bed an hour early tonight, then get up early tomorrow and do my aerobics tape tomorrow morning, perhaps adding ten extra minutes.

Negative thoughts:

- I'm so tired that I just can't move. I'm a failure at this exercise thing. I might as well just give it all up.
- I don't have time tonight to exercise. I'll never have time to fit in an exercise program.

Reward Yourself

In many aspects of our lives, we get rewards for the work we do. When we go to work each day, we come home with a paycheck. When we spend time and effort with our children, we are rewarded by seeing them grow and develop into happy, healthy, and productive people. If you adopt and maintain an exercise program, you deserve some rewards. The rewards should be what you value. You might find that the improved fitness and energy is reward enough for you. Or you may feel rewarded by losing enough fat that your dress size decreases by two sizes. You may like external rewards—you might want to reward yourself with a special vacation with a friend if you have met your fitness goals over the past six months. Many women reward themselves with food. Be careful that you do not reward yourself with calorie-dense foods. It can take a couple of hours to work off the calories in a piece of cake, for example. (See some examples of calorie exchanges between food and activities in Chapter 7.) The key is to figure out what you value and write down how you plan to reward yourself for your hard work!

Summary

- Make goals for yourself. A goal is realistic when it is specific, flexible, and measurable.
- Write down your exercise activities each day. Be diligent about this—it's the best way to keep track of what you're doing and how much progress you are making.
- Enlist your family and friends to help, and not hinder, you.
- Use problem solving to identify your challenges to exercise and to develop a plan to meet those challenges.
- Reward yourself!

17

Overcoming Fitness Roadblocks

Many things can interfere with your fitness goals. Some people call them excuses; we call them *fitness roadblocks*. From our clients and patients, we have heard just about every "reason" why someone cannot start or stick to an exercise program. (Many of these are ones we struggle with ourselves!) The problem is not motivation; most women are extremely motivated to lose weight and get in shape. The problems are that we let other life commitments get in our way and our attitudes prevent us from starting and sticking with an exercise program. The good news is that we have helped our clients and patients overcome their roadblocks. We have observed what works and what does not work. Now we are sharing this experience with you. This chapter presents several common fitness roadblocks. It helps you discover your fitness roadblocks and gives you tips on how to overcome them.

So often we hear, "If I could afford a personal trainer and someone to cook for me, I could lose weight like the movie stars." Millions of American women watch in awe as a television or movie star loses weight. The ones who manage to keep the weight off are those who adopt and maintain an exercise routine. The stars get the support they need by hiring personal trainers who prescribe a regular exercise and training program, give nutritional education and advice, and help them to organize their lives around their personal goals. The role of a personal trainer is to educate clients and help them to change their preconceived notions about exercise, nutrition, and themselves. You can be your own personal trainer by defining clear fitness goals for yourself, paying attention to what is getting in the way of your exercise program, and reading this book and others about diet and exercise. Being your own personal trainer means: first, deciding what are your goals for fitness; second, finding out what motivates you; and third, determining what is getting in the way of your goals. You have to be willing to analyze yourself in the context of your life and those around you. You must be willing to ask for support to accomplish your goals. And finally, you must be willing and committed to change.

Here are some common fitness roadblocks and some suggestions for overcoming them.

Tip for Breast Cancer Patients and Survivors

🖉 Many physical therapists and personal trainers are experts in therapeutic exercise and programs for special populations. Even if you do not feel you have any limitations following your cancer treatment or surgery, you may find it helpful to work with an exercise specialist who is knowledgeable about cancer rehabilitation.

🖉   "I Can't Afford to Join a Gym"

There are two possible scenarios here. The first is that you are on a very limited income and the cost of joining a gym is truly prohibitive for you. In this case, there are several alternatives. You can look into joining an inexpensive alternative. Local YWCA and YMCA clubs are well equipped and have very inexpensive joining fees and scholarships for low-income individuals and families. They are less likely to have trainers available, so you will need to read up on how to use equipment and, if possible, bring a friend with you who knows how to use the machines.

There are many ways to exercise that require a minimal investment of money to get started. Walking is one of the most effective ways of increasing fitness and burning calories, and the only thing you really need to get started is a comfortable and supportive pair of shoes! You could swim at a public pool. Most have adult-only hours where it is easier to do lap swimming. Most pools also provide swimming lessons for adults. Bicycling is inexpensive, especially if you buy a used bicycle. Check your paper's classified section. Many people purchase new bikes every few years and sell their hardly used ones at low cost.

The second possible scenario is that you can afford a club membership, but the cost looks too high to be worth it to you. If you put the cost in the context of your other monthly expenses, however, you may find that it is less expensive than you thought. Let's say you go for the big-city full-service gym and spend $75–$100 a month. If you divide that by 20 days a month, you have a cost of $4–$5 per day—about the cost of two double lattes. Not everyone needs the motivation of a gym to work out, however, and not everyone enjoys gym workouts. Decide what is your real reason for not wanting to put out the money for a health club membership. Pumping iron, sweating it out on a stair-stepper, or having to shower and see naked people you don't know may not be the way you want to spend your time. If a gym membership doesn't sound like a bargain to you, then take that money and allocate it monthly for something else that will get you closer to your fitness goal. Get a new exercise video, buy some walking/running gear, or purchase that bike you were going to buy last summer. Take a fitness vacation this year. There are a number of weekend camps and retreats that involve activities such as mountain biking or yoga, which can help jump-start your exercise program. Think of the money you are spending as an investment in your health and include this cost in your overall financial planning.

"I Don't Have Time to Exercise Because of My Travel Schedule"

Women who travel extensively for business or pleasure may find it challenging to exercise regularly. Always try to stay in a hotel that has a gym and/or pool. Be aware that the busiest times for the hotel gyms are usually early in the morning. You may have to plan to be at the facility as soon as it opens (and expect to find several other business travelers waiting with you). If your schedule is flexible, you could exercise before dinner or in the evening. If you do not like to vie for a space, however, you may be able to maintain your fitness level only by taking a walk during a meeting break or doing floor exercise in the hotel room. Doing *some* exercise while traveling is better than doing *none*. Maintaining some exercise while traveling will keep you from backsliding and losing what you gained while you were at home. Here are some ways to exercise while traveling.

- Opt for stairs and walking at airports, instead of escalators and moving sidewalks.
- While you are waiting for a flight, take a walk around the airport rather than sitting at the gate.
- Call ahead to your hotel to find out what kind of facilities they have. Some have VCRs available to rent, in which case you can bring an exercise tape to do in your room (or inquire if they have exercise tapes available).
- Bring resistive tubing, light dumbbells (under 5 pounds), or ankle weights with you to do exercises in your room. Bring travel weights that fill with water. You can find travel weights and other equipment suitable for travel in the back of travel magazines. Some business or upscale hotels are now providing exercise equipment in your room. Inquire about this when you make your reservations.
- Ask at the hotel registration or concierge desk for safe places to walk or run. Then fit in a walk or run before your meetings or at the end of the meeting day. Taking a walk in a new city is a great way to feel like you've had a little vacation break during your business trip.

If you cannot maintain your usual exercise program when traveling, your home exercise will need to be very consistent to balance the minimal exercise you do while away. The sample travel log below gives you an idea of how you can compensate for exercising less on the road. If you find it impossible to exercise while on a trip or to compensate when you are home, it may be time to reevaluate your travel schedule. Think about some possibilities for adapting your travel schedule so that you stop missing workouts. Or you might plan a day off every two or three weeks, just to catch up on your exercise and stay motivated. If getting in shape is a top priority, using your vacation days as "exercise days" may be the perfect solution to sticking with your exercise program. See Chapter 21 for more tips on fitting exercise into a busy schedule.

Table 17.1. Sample Exercise Program for Traveling

DAY	EXERCISE
Sunday home/travel	Stretching in hotel
Monday traveling	20-minute walk, abdominal exercise in hotel
Tuesday traveling	30-minute walk or hotel gym
Wednesday travel/home	no exercise
Thursday home	30-minute run, 30 minutes weights
Friday home	45-minute run
Saturday home	30-minute run, 30 minutes weights

Exercise Is Boring

Health clubs are packed with so many exercise choices these days that you never have to do the same workout twice. You also do not need to use the same mode of exercise for every workout to get results. For example, if you now use a stair-stepper three days a week, change to using the stair-stepper one day, a treadmill another day, and a rowing machine on the third day. Another option is a combination workout where you spend ten to twenty minutes on three different pieces of aerobic equipment. For example, you can do ten minutes on the stationary bike, ten minutes on the stair-stepper, and ten minutes on the treadmill, without any breaks in between.

Choose a workout regimen that you truly enjoy and eventually it won't feel like such "work." Did you know you burn more calories with in-line skating or line dancing (350 calories an hour) than you do walking for an hour (300 calories)? If you enjoy gardening, don't use electronic or motor-driven tools. Just use your own muscle power. You burn off about 300 calories per hour weeding, 350 calories per hour digging, and 400 calories per hour using a push mower.

If you find all types of exercise boring, the answer may be finding the right exercise partner rather than the right exercise. Having a walking partner makes the time fly by and helps you stick with your exercise schedule. Group exercise like walking clubs or exercise classes gives you social support and makes exercise more fun.

✐   "I Can't Exercise Until My Kids Are Older"

If you have a baby or toddler, use some of your time together outdoors walking or jogging. First, invest in a sturdy running stroller, which is more stable for brisk walking and running than a traditional baby stroller or carriage. If you have a tolerant baby or toddler, you can take your walk when she or he is awake. This way, you can enjoy the sights and sounds of the outdoors together. Taking your children with you while you exercise will also teach them that doing exercise and being fit are important and enjoyable parts of life. If your baby does not tolerate a stroller, use the baby's naptime to go for your walk. Just put her into the stroller and start walking. The movement will lull her to sleep, and you can get your exercise. Part of your fatigue as a new mother may be from not getting enough exercise, and you may find that you feel more energetic if you increase your fitness level.

✐   "I Hated Gym in School"

Many women were not encouraged as girls to be physically active, and their only experience with sports was in school physical education classes. Today, you have many more choices for physical fitness than you did in high school. Being good at sports is not required to be successful at exercise. Walking, running, and aerobic machines require very little coordination. However, if you would like to improve your skill in a sport or type of fitness, invest in a trainer who will teach you techniques and help build your confidence. Depending on where you live, a personal trainer will cost you about $35–$75 per hour. Another way to increase your coordination is to take an aerobics class at a community center or health club. The aerobics instructor can watch your technique and give you advice on how to make improvements.

If you are more interested in exercising your mind than your body, reconsider your exercise choices. Some intellectual types don't find exercise interesting. However, many forms of exercise can be very stimulating for the mind. Rock climbing, mountain biking, skiing, and racquet sports have been favorites among folks whose minds need stimulation to make exercise inviting. Tai chi and dance are additional options that can stimulate your mind and body. If your idea of recreation is to do needle-work, knitting, or other crafts and hobbies, promise yourself some quiet time with your hobby if you complete your exercise for the day. That way, you'll be rewarding yourself with your favorite activity.

"Being Overweight Runs in My Family"

If one or both of your parents were overweight or obese, you are also more likely to be overweight or obese. Part of this is because you have inherited your genetic blueprints from your parents. However the ten-dency to be sedentary and to have a poor diet is mostly learned rather than genetic. Exercising may be the best tool you have toward changing your metabolism and permanently improving your ability to keep off unwanted fat. Your family may not have provided exposure to sports or physical activity when you were growing up, which can make it difficult for you to take up these activities as an adult. Don't give up on your fam-ily, however. Perhaps one of them can be convinced to exercise with you. Someone in your immediate family who has had a similar upbringing and who really understands your struggles may make an excellent exercise buddy for you.

"The Only Reason I Am Trying to Lose Weight Is That My Husband Wants Me to Be Thinner"

If you are interested in becoming more fit only because your husband (or boyfriend, or parent, or children) wants you to lose weight, you will be less likely to succeed. Motivation needs to come from within in order for you to stick to your plan. Everyone needs some kind of motivation to stick with an exercise program and lose weight. Motivation comes in various forms, such as wanting to look good in a bathing suit this summer, or wanting to look good for your twenty-year high school reunion. It is appro-priate to want to please your significant other and to stay healthy out of respect for your life together. However, don't let your physical appearance be "one of the problems" of your relationship with your husband or part-ner. If including your partner in your exercise plan is important to you, be specific about what kind of help you want from that person. If it doesn't help you to be criticized when you skip your morning walk or have a second piece of cake, make it clear that you do not want that kind of feedback. Talk with your family, friends, and loved ones about what does work for you. You need their support in order for your exercise plan to work smoothly, but the key ingredient to your success is you.

"I Don't Look Good in Exercise Clothes"

If you are like most women, you are concerned about how you look in workout gear and you wouldn't be caught dead in spandex. We have found that many women are modest and having to wear so little makes them uncomfortable even if they don't have a lot of fat to lose. Don't worry—you do not need to wear spandex in order to work out. You just need to wear comfortable, breathable clothing. Look for clothes made from breathable synthetic fabric, which allows sweat to evaporate and keeps you feeling cooler. If you are doing high-intensity exercise, you may be more comfortable in shorts and a short-sleeve shirt, but the shorts can be long so that you do not feel like you are baring too much. Outdoor clothing stores carry a variety of lightweight pants and shorts that make exercising outdoors more comfortable. There are several mail-order catalogs that carry workout athletic clothing that are specially designed for women's bodies. If you are very uncomfortable wearing exercise clothing, you could opt to exercise at home or at an all-women's gym. With time and a little trial and error you'll find what feels best.

Tip for Breast Cancer Patients and Survivors

If you have had a mastectomy without reconstruction and prefer to exercise without your prosthesis, you may find it more comfortable to go to a women-only gym rather than to a coed gym. In general, women-only health clubs are fairly inexpensive and have a number of classes especially designed for women. You might also want to consider attending a retreat for breast cancer survivors that focuses on wellness.

"I've Tried Everything but I Can't Find an Exercise Program That Works"

Do you really believe that the right exercise program just has not come along yet? To meet your goals, you must make sure that there is a match between the type of exercise you have chosen and the plan you have devised. If you want to lose weight and improve cardiovascular fitness, brisk walking or running can meet your goal. If you want to increase your strength and muscle mass, weight lifting will be a critical part of your exercise plan. How often and how long you exercise are as important to getting results as how hard you exercise. No matter what form of exercise you choose, you must be consistent in order to see results. Perhaps you have a hard time sticking to your current program. Before you give up on exercise, look for a better exercise video, gym, or walking group, evaluate the effectiveness of your program, and make sure that you have set goals and matched your program to those goals. (See Chapter 14 for more information on how to add an exercise plan to your life.)

"I Have Back Problems"

Back pain, especially lower-back pain, is one of the most common complaints of women. Much of this pain is caused by a combination of improper lifting, poor back and abdominal muscle strength, and tight muscles. There are a variety of ways to increase abdominal tone. Abdominal crunches are a safer and more effective way to strengthen the abdominal muscles than are the old-fashioned full sit-ups. A toned abdomen also comes from getting the deep muscles of the abdomen active. Using the abdominal muscles all day long increases abdominal muscle tone. When you are unloading the dishwasher, taking out the garbage, or sitting at a meeting, use your abdominal muscles by pulling the "belly button to spine." This contracts the deep muscles and supports your back. You can also work your abdominal muscles during aerobic exercise and sports. Learning to involve and integrate your abdominal muscles into activities like cycling and tennis not only improves the look of your midsection but also improves your skill at the sport. Using your abdominal muscles while weight training is another way to increase abdominal tone. During your weight-lifting session, squeeze the abdominal muscles in as you push or pull the weight. This contracts the abdominal muscles, leading to improved strength, and it teaches your body to use your abdominal muscles during physical movement.

However, low-back pain can also be caused by tightness in the back muscles and decreased range of motion surrounding joints. A regular stretching program for your back as well as hips and legs will aid in preventing increased pain while exercising. Be sure to check with your doctor or physical therapist before beginning back exercises if you have pain. For more information and exercise for abdominal reconditioning and back stretching, see Chapter 19.

Tip for Breast Cancer Patients and Survivors

.✐ It is safe for women who have had breast or reconstructive surgery to do crunches, but the time you must wait after your surgery may vary. Some types of surgery could limit your choices for abdominal exercise. Be sure to consult with your surgeon prior to starting an abdominal regimen. See Chapter 19 for more information about doing abdominal exercise following breast surgery.

✐   "Whenever I Exercise, I Hurt Something"

You went hiking with your friends three days ago. You climbed steadily uphill for three hours, then downhill for two hours. Suffice it to say that this is not the usual way you spend your day. You felt a little sore at the end of the day. The next morning you woke up in agony. Your legs were killing you. Your back and neck were stiff. All you wanted to do was to stay in bed all day, but you had to get up and go to work. A few days later you are still feeling sore, although its getting better. If you frequently experience considerable pain after exercise, the most likely reason is that you have pushed yourself too far too fast. While sore muscles are inevitable if you push yourself hard enough, you can minimize your risk by progressing slowly toward your goal. A good rule of thumb is to increase your exercise by 10 percent each workout. For example, start by walking the track ten laps (2¼ miles). In your next workout, increase 10 percent by walking 2½ miles. We described goals and exercise progression further in Chapters 15 and 16.

Summary

- There are many "roadblocks" to starting and maintaining a regular exercise program. The good news is that these roadblocks can all be overcome in one way or another.
- You need support in order to overcome your fitness roadblocks. Your most important supporter is yourself—you can be your own fitness trainer. Other support can come from family, friends, and coworkers.
- To overcome your roadblocks you must first decide what are your fitness goals, what motivates you, and what is getting in the way of your goals.
- There is an exercise program that fits into any busy lifestyle. Exercise does not have to be expensive, flashy, or complicated. You don't have to be an athlete to increase your level of exercise. It can be done at home or when you travel. It can be as exciting as you want to make it. You can exercise on your own, with your children, with your husband, with family, or with friends.
- Exercise can help reduce stress in your life and can help you adopt other healthy behaviors. As a result, you will feel better and will have more energy to exercise.

18

Strength Training

The average American woman loses between seven and ten pounds of muscle between age twenty-five and forty. Most of this muscle loss is from not using muscles rather than something that inevitably happens with aging. The adage "use it or lose it" is true for your muscles. When you go on a diet, you usually lose muscle mass along with fat. Weight training is one way of ensuring that you retain as much muscle as possible. In this chapter we describe why you should add a strength-training program to your exercise regimen. We give you some information on muscle biology. We provide information about the different types of strength training. Finally, we give tips to help you start and maintain a strength-training program.

Why You Should Increase Your Muscle Strength and Mass

Your body is composed primarily of muscle, bone, water, and fat. Muscle burns more calories than does fat. If you have more muscle, your metabolism works at a higher rate. Your *metabolism* determines how fast you use calories and how many calories you need to accomplish your daily activities.

Weight lifting, particularly free weights, strengthens your postural

Tip for Breast Cancer Patients and Survivors

~~*~~   After a breast cancer diagnosis, women have a tendency to lose muscle due to months or years of treatment and inactivity. Rebuilding muscle is key to a successful cancer rehabilitation and recovery program. Increased muscle improves energy reserves, decreases fatigue, and helps manage pain. Most important, the strength you gain enhances your ability to do the daily activity that you currently find difficult, such as throwing the ball for your dog, doing yard work, or returning to a physically demanding occupation.

muscles, which stabilize your body during movement. Postural muscles include the abdominal and back muscles.

Women in our culture have a tendency to slouch. Chronic slouching weakens back and abdominal muscles. If you slouch, your body gets accustomed to the slouched position so that sitting upright is exhausting. Weight lifting, with proper form, strengthens muscles into the erect position. You can condition your back muscles, which can result in a taller posture, by paying attention to your postural muscles during your weight-training sessions. You will find that during weight lifting you naturally want sit or stand taller to adequately move the weights. It takes some practice, but with just a few weight training-sessions you will find it less comfortable to slouch and more comfortable to hold yourself upright. Increasing your overall body strength can be a very powerful tool.

Wouldn't it be nice to be able to help move your furniture around or not worry how heavy your grocery bags are? Having a stronger body will help keep you from being injured while doing basic life chores. Many occupations can lead to overuse of certain muscles throughout the day, leaving other muscles relatively unused and weakened. This is how muscle imbalances develop that can lead to occupational injuries. A well thought out weight-training program can help to compensate for this imbalance.

To summarize, strength training can help you to lose fat mass and keep lean, which may be important in reducing risk for breast cancer after menopause. It can help you maintain an aerobic exercise program by strengthening muscles so that your joints and tendons can better tolerate the stresses of exercise. Finally, it improves your posture and increases your capacity for strength-requiring chores, which will help to reduce risk of injuries. Avoiding injuries will help you to keep on a steady exercise program for life.

Measuring Your Muscle Mass

Your *body composition* can be measured as the percentages of your body that are composed of fat mass and lean mass. Lean mass is a combination of muscle, connective tissue, bone, fluids, and everything else that makes up your body except fat. If you are 25 percent body fat, you are 75 percent lean mass. Many fitness enthusiasts are now measuring their percent body fat in addition to measuring their weight. This can be done with a technique called bioelectric impedance. Most gyms have bioelectric impedance machines or equipment that measures body composition. You can also purchase a home version of the bioelectric impedance for about $100. When evaluating your body composition, be sure to look at how much lean mass you have as well as how much fat. If you lose muscle, your percent fat will go up. If you lose fat, your percent lean mass will go up. If you do not have access to a bioelectric impedance machine, you can measure your muscle progress by first noticing increases in strength and second by noticing results in the mirror.

How Muscles Grow

When you develop muscle mass, you are not actually growing more muscle cells. Each muscle fiber or cell is made of tiny strands called myofibrils. When you regularly exercise your muscles, these myofibrils expand and eventually give the muscle a more toned, smooth look. When you challenge your muscles with weight training, these myofibrils expand even more than they do with aerobic activity like running. If you run a lot, your legs become toned. If you do weight lifting, your legs become more toned and developed, and they do so at a faster rate than with aerobic activity. In general, you will feel increases in strength after about six weeks of a consistent weight-training program. You will see increase in muscle tone and size in about twelve weeks. The increased strength in the first six weeks of a weight-training program comes from improved coordination and more efficient movement.

✍ Muscle Growth in Women Compared with Muscle Growth in Men

Men can build very large muscles with weight training because they have large amounts of testosterone. Testosterone is an anabolic hormone. That means that it helps to build up body tissues. Since women have lower amounts of testosterone, they do not build very large muscles with weight training. All women have some testosterone in their bodies, but some women naturally produce more than others do. Men have about twenty to thirty times more testosterone than do women. Men also have about 30 percent more muscle mass in their lower body and about 50 percent more muscle mass in their upper body, compared with women. They have the ability to develop more muscle partly because they are starting out with more muscle mass to begin with. This is one theory of why men seem to be able to eat more and not gain weight. They have more muscle to fuel; therefore their metabolism is set at a higher rate and they burn off more calories when they exercise.

A common fear among women is that if they lift weights they will get too big, even as large as a bodybuilder. The good news is that very few women have the ability to build large, bulky muscle. This can be frustrating for competitive women who do want to develop their muscles. Even if you have a body type that "bulks up" with weight training, you can control the amount of muscle growth. The amount of muscle mass increase is related to the type of weight-training regimen. Overdevelopment of muscles will happen only with specific, intense training. For example, you could become very muscular and bulky with weight training for twelve to fifteen hours each week. You can become stronger and have more muscle definition, however, with just three to five hours of weight training a week. This amount of training will not make you bulky.

✒ Types of Weight-Training Equipment

There are four basic types of weight equipment you will run across at a gym or a retail store. The name brand or package may look different, but the mechanism and design are the same. The most important difference among the types of equipment is how they cause your muscles to respond and perform.

Equipment with a Pulley System

A pulley system is one of the oldest forms of machines. In this system, a weight is pulled by cable around a circular pulley. Pulley machines are low maintenance and inexpensive. The weight amount on a pulley system is the same throughout the range of motion of a muscle contraction. You will find that the weight is easier to lift at some points of the range and more difficult at others. This is because your muscles are more efficient in some positions than in others. You will notice that your muscle contractions vary in response to the weight.

Machines with a Vary Weight System

A vary weight system uses a pulley to move the weight, but the resistance changes as the weight moves through the range of motion. Unlike the original pulley, this new system increases weight when the lift becomes easier and decreases it when the lift is more difficult. When you use this system, you will notice that the weight feels the same at all positions. Fitness experts believe that this type of system trains muscles in a more thorough and effective manner compared to a simple pulley system. Many manufacturers have developed similar systems that adjust the weight amounts to your efforts without your being aware of the adjustments.

Machines with a Hydraulic System

There are a variety of hydraulic weight-training machines that use hydraulic pistons to control the weight. The harder or faster you push or pull the weight, the harder the weight becomes to move. The resistance changes in response to your muscular velocity. These machines are popular with athletes who play contact sports. When you use one of these machines, you get the feeling that it is pushing back as you push the weight. Hydraulics can be very effective in helping heal muscles that can't handle a lot of dead weight but respond well to gradual increases in resistance.

Tip for Breast Cancer Patients and Survivors

✍ Following breast surgery and/or reconstruction, it may be safer to begin exercise on machines rather than with free weights. The support of the machine helps extremely deconditioned women who do not have enough strength in their trunk to support their body movements with the free weights. On a machine, the abdominal, back, and shoulder muscles do not work as hard. However, for a women with less muscle dysfunction after surgery, using free weights (as low as 1 pound) helps bring back abdominal tone and improves overall muscle balance. Posture is also improved with free weights. Women who have had a mastectomy may have a tendency to slouch more and need to pay closer attention to their posture. Sometimes the tendency to slouch comes from the tightness that has developed in the chest due to the surgery. Stretching the chest and shoulder muscles and strengthening the back muscles remedies this imbalance and improves posture.

Free Weights

Free weights are simple, straightforward equipment. The weight stays the same from beginning to end of the movement. There are several types of free weight, including benches, racks, bars, and dumbbells. Working with free weights resembles lifting weight in the real world. In the real world, you pick up a box and you put it down; you do not have pulleys and hydraulics to help support your movement. With free weight equipment, the weight is a set resistance that doesn't change as you move it. A 5-pound dumbbell is a 5-pound dumbbell from the start of the lift to the end.

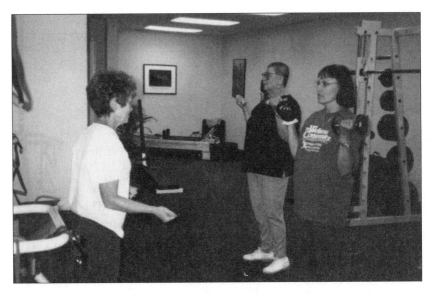

Working with free weights maximizes the use of the trunk muscles: abdomen, back, chest, and buttocks. Women doing biceps curls with free weights at Indoor Training, a program sponsored by Team Survivor California. Photo by Team Survivor Califorina. Photo: Karen Van Kirk.

The Benefits of Free Weights

You may find the thought of working with free weights intimidating. There are a number of benefits to working with free weights, however, that may make it worth your while to overcome your fear or hesitation.

Free Weights Increase Use of
Abdomen, Back, Chest, and Buttocks

Your body as a whole works harder during a free-weight exercise than with the same exercise on a machine. When you do a biceps curl while standing or sitting, your shoulder girdle, back, and abdomen are all working to keep the body stable so that you can move the weight efficiently. This is important for improvement in endurance, strength, and muscle tone of the back, chest, abdomen, and buttocks. Although some free-weight exercises, such as the chest press or leg press, are done with the support of a bench, you can get a complete workout standing or sitting on a stool to maximize use of the trunk muscles.

Tip for Breast Cancer Patients and Survivors

✐ In women at risk, weight lifting can trigger a lymphedema response. Although strong muscles can improve lymph flow, you should use caution with weight training. General weight-lifting exercises for the upper body may be performed safely with light weights. Use 1- to 3-pound dumbbells to start. Be sure to monitor your upper body closely for any swelling as you increase weight and repetitions. Lymphedema-sensitive weight-lifting exercises improve upper body strength and lymph flow. If you are concerned about lymphedema or already have lymphedema, be sure to consult your surgeon or oncologist, or a physical therapist who specializes in lymphedema before beginning a weight-lifting program. For more information about lymphedema, see Chapter 9.

Free Weights Improve Posture

Posture is important for health as well as appearance. After years of slouching it becomes exhausting to sit up straight and maintain that stance. Try it. Lift your chest and pull your shoulders back, and after just a couple of minutes you feel fatigued. Your muscles want to go back to their slouching posture where they are more comfortable because that has become their strongest position. Proper use of free weights enhances posture by strengthening your muscles in an erect position. Eventually slouching becomes less comfortable, and sitting and standing taller are more natural and comfortable postures.

It is common to notice strength before you notice any changes in your muscle definition or tone. The strength changes in the first six weeks are a result of your repetition and practice with the weights. You become better at controlling the weights and therefore can lift more weight. It takes about twelve weeks before actual muscle tone occurs.

Free Weights Provide Physical and Mental Variety

If you find weight training boring, you may prefer working with free weights. Free-weight training is more stimulating than some of the weight-training machines. There are a number of different free-weight exercises for each muscle group, so you can create a variety of exercise

Figure 18.1. Strength and muscle changes over twelve weeks of weight training

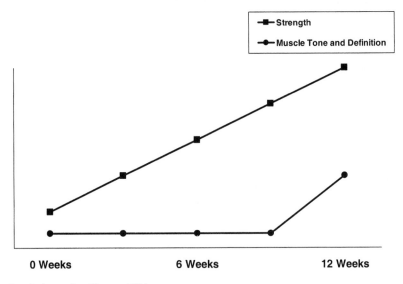

Graph design by Clayton Hibbert.

routines. Although the exercises are different in each routine, the muscles receive the same workout. Many fitness specialists believe that doing a variety of exercises for each muscle group improves the effectiveness of a weight-training routine. For example, there are at least four different biceps exercises using a curl bar, straight bar, dumbbell, and preacher bench. Each exercise puts a different demand on the biceps and other arm muscles, which improves the overall tone of the arm. Although you see many bodybuilders using free weights, this does not mean that free-weight equipment develops bigger muscles. People who do want to develop mass prefer free weights because with the variety of exercises they can put higher demands on their muscles, which increases their chances of better muscle growth. In one workout, someone wanting to increase her arm size may do six different exercises for the arm muscles. This repetitive workload to the arm exhausts the muscles more thoroughly and accelerates development of the arm muscles.

Free Weights Are Inexpensive and Accessible

Most free-weight equipment is inexpensive and accessible. Handheld dumbbells are manufactured in various sizes and sold by the pound. In a large sporting goods store they may cost as little as 75¢ to $1 per pound. A pair of 2-pound weights, therefore, cost about $4. A good set includes 1-, 2-, and 5-pound weights. (You can double up to get 3, 6, and 7 pounds.) If you have never worked with free weights, start with 1- and 2-pound dumbbells for upper-body strengthening. As your muscles get stronger, increase the weights. Always keep your lighter weights close at hand, as you may need to drop back down to lighter weights at some point because of illness or long lapses in your weight-training program. If you have done some weight training before, then you may be able to begin with 3- and 5-pound weights. You should own at least three different size pairs of weights to do an effective home weight-training program.

Combining Free Weights and Machines Can Be Ideal

All of the types of weight equipment that we have discussed are appropriate and effective for strength training in women. Most women prefer a combination of free weights and machines to add variety and to create the most effective program for their goals. There are some exercises that you cannot do effectively with free weights. For example, it is very difficult to isolate the hamstring muscles and pull an effective amount of weight using free weights. These muscles are better trained on a hamstring machine because the leg is stabilized and the hamstring muscles can be isolated. As you work with weights, you will learn which exercises you like better on machines and which exercises you like better with free weights. The most important thing to remember is that *all* weight-training equipment is effective. Use the equipment that you like: If you like it, you will do it!

Creating Your Own Weight-Training Program

When you start learning about strength training, you will find that there are many different recipes for the same results. Choosing the number of sets, repetitions, and workouts per week is all part of designing your training program. The first question that you should ask yourself is what results you want from your weight lifting. Are you looking for more strength in your muscles to lift heavy luggage? Are you hoping for more tone and definition? Are you strength training for a specific sport like rock climbing? Do you want more power in your tennis serve? Weight-training results are directly related to how you train. Strength, endurance, and power all can be accomplished with weight training when done appropriately for your goals. The second important question to ask yourself is how much time you want to spend every week lifting weights. Do you want to spend two hours each week? How about six hours? You also must consider travel time to the gym if that is where you choose to do your weight routine. If you don't have the time to dedicate to it, you won't do the program and you won't get results. Is it easier for you to go the gym six days a week and stay for thirty minutes, or do you prefer to go three days each for ninety minutes at a time? Each exercise will take you about three to five minutes, unless you are lifting heavy weights and need more break time. A thirty-minute workout with warm-up and stretching allows enough time for about eight weight-training exercises and

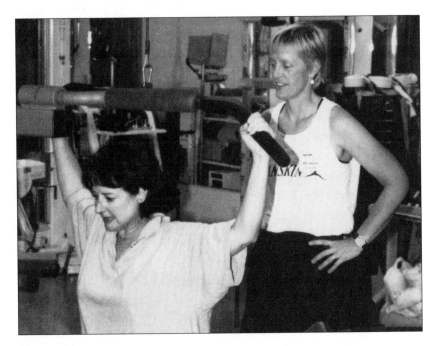

The support of a trainer can help you increase your weight safely and help you set goals. Vicki Boehman and trainer Michelle Kunzwiler at Indoor Training, sponsored by Team Survivor Northwest in Seattle.

a basic overall conditioning program. Once you have a clear goal and have committed the time to attain it, you can start designing your weight-lifting program.

In our recommendations below, we give some standard programs with a specific number of times an exercise is repeated. Exercise experts now believe that exercising muscles until they are fatigued, rather than a pre-specified number, is more effective in weight training. However, weight training to fatigue should be done only with a training partner or the help of a personal trainer working with you as you exercise. If you do this on your own, you are at significant risk of injuring yourself. If you plan to start a weight-training program on your own, therefore, we recommend that you use the more standard regimens that we have given you below.

Repetitions, Sets, and Frequency

Weight training is done with sets and repetitions. A *repetition* (or "rep") is one lift and lowering of the weight. The total times you lift and lower the weight is a set. Your goals will determine the number of repetitions that should be in each set. It is more important in the beginning to consider how many reps you are going to do than how much weight you are going to lift. The most common routine is three sets of ten reps. A set of ten reps gives a balance between strength and endurance.

If you want to add muscle mass, do fewer reps with more weight. If you are looking for endurance, then do more repetitions using less weight. The amount of weight is gauged by the number of repetitions. For example, if you are weight training to condition your legs for cross-country running, then you would perhaps do six sets of twenty reps. If you are training for rock climbing, then you would lift in short sets, such as two sets of six reps. As you can see with these two extremes, three sets of ten falls somewhere in between to give you some strength and some endurance. When deciding the number of sets, you need to think of your goals. If power and strength are your main goals, two to three sets should be enough. If you want to increase endurance, then four to six sets is a more effective choice. Below are some examples of reps and sets that yield certain goals. Coaches and trainers have many regimens they pre-scribe for specific results. You can see how the number of repetitions and sets naturally monitors how much weight you can use.

Table 18.1. Repetitions and Sets to Attain Certain Goals

GOAL	SETS AND REPS	AMOUNT OF WEIGHT
Endurance	5 sets of 20 reps *or* 6 sets of 25 reps	Very light weight
Weight loss	3 sets of 20 reps *or* 4 sets of 25 reps	Light weight
General tone	2 sets of 15 reps *or* 3 sets of 10 reps *or* 4 sets of 12 reps	Average weight
Strength	3 sets of 10 reps *or* 3 sets of 8 reps	Heavy weight

Endurance

Endurance means being able to do something for a longer period of time. Whether walking, skiing, or lifting repetitive boxes at work, you build endurance by doing more repetitions and using lighter weight. For you to be able to do five sets of twenty reps or six sets of twenty-five reps, the weight must be light enough that you can complete all the sets and repetitions without failure. In fact, from the first set to the last, the weight should be manageable and you should not have to strain. The difference is how much time you have to do a endurance-enhancing regime; six sets of twenty-five reps will take you longer to complete but yield results a bit faster.

If you are interested in conditioning for a certain sport, you should do what is called "sport specific" exercises. This means doing exercise that mimics the motions you do during your sport activity. For example, lunges are good leg strengtheners for runners and hikers. Pull-down machines help increase the power in the upper body for rock climbers. Some sport-oriented clubs have equipment that is designed for a specific sport. One example is a swim machine, where you lie prone and "swim" freestyle with pulleys in your hands. Of course it is not exactly like swimming, but the more specific you can make your weight training the more your sport performance benefits. Endurance programs need to be done at least three days a week or every other day to yield results.

Weight Loss

Many overweight women have the misconception that they need to lose all of their extra fat *before* beginning a weight-training program. As we have discussed previously, including weights in your exercise plans during weight loss improves your chances of losing more fat and retaining more muscle. One standard protocol for weight loss is three sets of twenty reps or four sets of twenty-five reps. Your sets should not feel stressful; the weight you use should be fairly comfortable from the first repetition to the last. Keeping the number of repetitions fairly high increases time that the muscles are worked, which sends a message to the brain and muscle system that the skeletal muscles are in demand. This helps to maintain a higher and consistent level of muscle mass. A higher level of muscle mass sets you up for a more successful fat-loss program. This type of weight training should be done every other day without more than two days in between at any time.

Using Circuit Training in Your Weight-Loss Program

To burn fat, your body needs to be operating in an aerobic state. If weight loss is your goal, you may want to start a weight-training program that is fairly aerobic. One way to do this is with an aerobic circuit workout. In a circuit workout, you go from station to station quickly and do not take a very long break in between weight-training exercises. You do two weight-training exercises and then five minutes on an aerobic machine. You repeat this so that at the end you have done all of your weight-training exercises with a short break of aerobic exercise in between. The example below would take about an hour and fifteen minutes because it includes a twenty-minute final aerobic segment. If you choose to do just aerobic exercise on alternate days, then this circuit would take less than an hour.

The aerobic weights circuit is a popular routine for women who do not have a lot of time but want to increase their aerobic capacity and improve their overall muscle tone and are concerned with weight management. If you do this at a gym, we caution that during peak gym hours it may be difficult to get access repeatedly to the aerobic equipment. A circuit workout for losing fat should be done every other day or three times a week for best results. If you prefer more than three exercise sessions each week, it is safe to do this regimen two on and one off. This means you exercise two days in a row and then take a day off. If you *still* do not want that day off, you need to substitute another form of exercise that is less taxing on your muscles, such as walking or swimming, to avoid an overuse injury.

Sample Aerobic Circuit Training Workout with Weights

- Abdominal exercise
- Leg press
- Stair-stepper, five minutes
- Chest press
- Shoulder press
- Bike, five minutes
- Front lifts
- Lateral lifts
- Stair-stepper, five minutes
- Lat pull down
- Seated row
- Bike, five minutes
- Biceps curls
- Triceps extensions
- Treadmill walk, twenty minutes

General Muscle Tone

For overall general toning, we have listed a few different options in Table 18-1. The best choice for you depends on how much time you have and what feels right to you. You may want to choose fewer sets and more reps if you have a short attention span. Some research suggests that fewer sets with more reps is just as effective as the standard three sets of ten reps regime. Some specialists even suggest that one set of reps will give you the same results as three sets of ten. Be sure that the last few repetitions of each set are somewhat challenging. If the weight feels fairly comfortable and requires more effort by the end of the set, you are at the right weight to increase your muscle tone. The only way to discover what works for you is to try different regimes and then tailor your program by what fits in best to your schedule, what you feel is giving you the results you want, and what you enjoy. It is best to do a general toning program

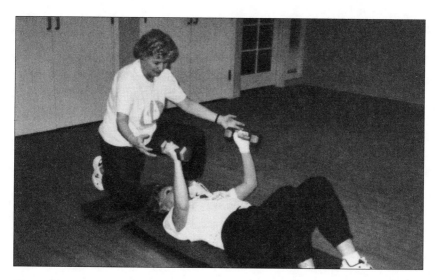

Karin Queen spotting Sue Dickens as she does a chest press with free weights. When lifting heavy weights to the point of muscle fatigue, it is important to use a "spotter." Photo: Lisa Talbott.

every other day, or three to four days a week. Results are quicker if you can keep up this number of workouts per week. But don't get too inflexible! For example, if you usually do your weight training on Monday, Wednesday, and Friday, and you are going out of town for the weekend, work out Thursday instead. Two days in a row is perfectly fine if you are not lifting heavy weights and putting very high demands on your muscles.

Strength

To increase your muscle strength, you need to exercise to the point of fatigue. This means that you lift until you simply cannot do one more repetition. If you are using free weights, this can be dangerous without a spotter during some exercises. The weight must be heavy enough so that by the end of the set you are struggling and have difficulty finishing the last two or three repetitions. Stressing the muscles this way breaks down the muscle tissue, allowing it to build back stronger. It is important to increase your weight slowly so that you do not injure your joints or strain your muscles. Using a weight belt will decrease strain on your lower back.

Increase weight gradually and with careful thought. Careful thought

Tip for Breast Cancer Patients and Survivors

Increase weight and repetitions gradually. Following cancer treatment or surgery, you may find that starting with a short set, such as one set of five reps, is the most comfortable amount of lifting. You can then gradually increase repetition using a light weight, until you reach a more effective regime, such as three sets of twelve repetitions. Be sure to talk with your surgeon if you have had surgery to your axillary lymph nodes before doing upper-body weight training.

This is a sensible schedule for increasing your weight training:

1 set of 5 reps
2 sets of 5 reps
3 sets of 5 reps
3 sets of 7 reps
3 sets of 10 reps
3 sets of 12 reps

Increase repetitions every two or three consistent weight-lifting sessions. Once you are comfortable with three sets of twelve reps at a specific weight, increase weight slowly, every three to four workouts. After increasing the weight, you may need to decrease repetitions and build back up to the original three sets of twelve reps. Or, rather than using the same weight for all three sets, use a heavier weight for the first set and then a lighter weight for the following two sets. This is a safe way to work up gradually to using the heavier weight for all three sets.

	SET 1	SET 2	SET 3
Week 1	2 pounds/12 reps	2 pounds/12 reps	2 pounds/12 reps
Week 2	3 pounds/12 reps	2 pounds/12 reps	2 pounds/12 reps
Week 3	3 pounds/12 reps	3 pounds/12 reps	2 pounds/12 reps
Week 4	3 pounds/12 reps	3 pounds/12 reps	3 pounds/12 reps

means you *must* keep a log and pay close attention to each and every workout. If you miss a workout and do not recall where you left off the last time, you are more likely to hurt yourself. You also should do flexibility exercises and get plenty of rest between workouts to decrease your chances of injury. When you work your muscles to the point of fatigue, you should rest them for forty-eight hours before your next workout. (This just means no weight training on that particular muscle for forty-eight hours; it does not mean that you should lie down for forty-eight hours!) Women who like to work out often might do upper-body exercises three days per week and lower-body exercises on the other three days to allow muscles to rest between workouts.

Body Sculpting

Body sculpting is the process of using weights to change the shape and form of your body. You tailor your weight-training regimen to match your specific body type. There are three basic body types for women: "pear," "apple," and "general." Your body type may change with age or as you lose fat, so it's important to review your shape every few years.

For a general toning program that will also give you more muscle definition, fitness specialists commonly recommend three sets of ten reps of each exercise, three days a week. To change your body shape, slim down some areas, and increase muscle in others, however, you need to match your weight-training exercises to your specific goals. Not every exercise needs to be the same number of repetitions. If you have a pear-shaped figure and you want to trim your lower body and broaden your shoulders, you might do weights, three sets of eight reps on the shoulders using heavier weights, and three sets of fifteen reps for the lower body with an intermediate amount of weight. It is just as important to do muscle-building upper-body exercises when sculpting a pear-shaped figure as the reducing lower-body exercises if your goal is to change your body's proportions. If you are more barrel-shaped, you should do the opposite sculpting regimen to build up thin legs and reduce the upper body. It is sometimes difficult to analyze your own body type. You might talk with a trainer at your gym or with a nutritionist to help clarify your body type. Or see Appendix A for hints on how to determine your body shape.

Eating to Fuel Your Weight-Training Workouts

Your eating plan need not vary greatly because of your new interest in a weight-training program. Some specialists believe that if you weight-train you should eat more protein. This may be true when doing a muscle-building program. However, for all of the programs we have discussed thus far, a balanced diet with about 50 grams of protein a day is sufficient to repair muscle tissue and maintain proper muscle cell metabolism. The biggest secret to a leaner physique that many weight-training enthusiasts do not realize is that the quality of what you eat plays a large part in the success of your program. Muscle definition and a leaner look are gained by maintaining a healthy diet (not too many calories and minimizing fats and simple sugars) and losing fat in and around the muscles. Since aerobic exercise is the best way to burn fat, be sure to maintain a regular aerobic program along with your weight-training sessions every week. Do not fall into the trap of spending so much time with your weight-training program that you do not allow enough time to keep up with your aerobic exercise.

Summary

- The loss of muscle mass with aging is not inevitable and can be prevented and reversed with appropriate strength-training exercises.
- Dieting or any other weight loss without exercise results in considerable loss of muscle along with fat and water.
- Your percent body fat may be a better measure to gauge progress than your weight. If you do not have access to a bioelectric impedance measure, you can measure the circumference of your waist and hips.
- Muscles need more energy in the form of calories than do other body components, such as fat. If your muscles increase in size, you will burn more of the calories you take in.
- Weight training helps to improve posture and to stabilize delicate areas such as knee joints.
- When you start a weight-training program, you will feel stronger within six weeks, and you will see differences in muscle tone and definition within twelve weeks.
- Your choice of a weight-training program depends on whether you want to concentrate on strength, endurance, tone and definition, preparation for a specific sport, fat loss, or balance.

19

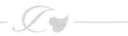

Conditioning Exercises

Conditioning exercises strengthen your muscles, stabilize your joints, and improve exercise performance. Aerobic exercise is enhanced when muscles are flexible and strong and joints are well supported. In this chapter we present a variety of ways to improve the health of your muscles and joints.

Relaxation, Meditation, and Breathing

Relaxation is sometimes all that tight muscles need to reduce pain and injury. You may find that your muscles relax if you practice daily meditation. Focused relaxation of the muscles through meditation can reduce pain and improve emotional well-being. Positive visualization from meditation can also improve your exercise performance.

Diaphragmatic breathing is another way to relax tense muscles. The diaphragm, a domelike muscle that forms the floor of the rib cage, is the most efficient muscle for breathing and relaxation. Correct diaphragmatic breathing can help to quiet brain activity, resulting in the relaxation of all the muscles and organs of the body. This is accomplished by slow, rhythmic breathing concentrated in the diaphragm rather than the chest. This breathing technique can be done first thing in the morning before you get out of bed, or at night before you fall asleep. Diaphragmatic

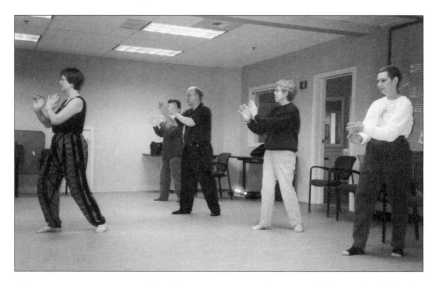

Qi gong is an ancient art form that encourages relaxation of the mind and body. It can be done in a group or alone. Pictured is a qi gong class at Cancer Lifeline in Seattle, Washington. Photo: Doris Wong-Estridge.

breathing can also be used prior to your exercise session and can be done lying down, sitting, or standing. Diaphragmatic breathing can ease the daily stress of your day. When things get hectic at work or home, stop, take a few deep diaphragmatic breaths, and relax. Many meditation and relaxation techniques are just as helpful when done in small periods throughout the day as when done for one longer session.

To Do Diaphragmatic Breathing

- Place both hands on your abdomen
- Exhale completely through the mouth, allowing your abdomen and chest to fall.
- Inhale deeply though the nose while contracting your diaphragm. It will move downward, causing your abdomen to rise. Keep your chest and shoulders relaxed during this exercise.
- Breathe slowly—don't force your breathing.
- Repeat until you feel your muscles and mind relax. Most women report that they feel best after doing three sets of five breaths with a few regular breaths in between for a break.

✍ Flexibility and Mobility

Stretching helps to prevent injury to your muscles and joints. Maintaining flexibility decreases your chances of a muscle strain while exercising. When your joints are well supported by strong, agile muscles, you are less apt to injure yourself. Flexibility helps your body adapt to stressful situations and decreases your chance of injury. For example, if you unexpectedly step down off a curb while running, flexible muscles will absorb the jarring motion. If your muscles are tight, a sudden stress could cause a strain. Mobility and range of motion of your joints decrease naturally with age. However, you can maintain mobility by daily stretching exercises. Overuse is better managed when muscles are stretched and allowed to relax and rejuvenate. A daily stretching program will help to reduce your chances of developing problems in your neck, lower back, knees, and other joints.

Guidelines for a Daily Stretch Program

- Your stretching environment should be calm, relaxing and comfortable.
- A general five-minute warm-up such as walking, marching in place, or light dancing should be performed prior to stretch-

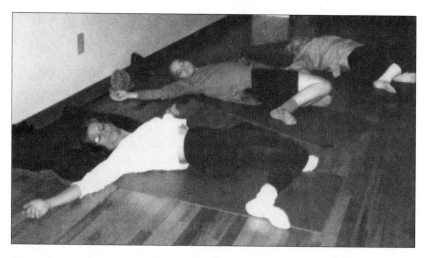

Yoga is an excellent way to relax and stretch tense muscles. Pictured is a yoga class sponsored by Cancer Lifeline, in Seattle, Washington. Photo: Lisa Talbott.

Tip for Breast Cancer Patients and Survivors

✐ If you have regained full range of motion in your upper body and mobility of your shoulders since your breast or reconstruction surgery, the suggested daily stretch is safe for you to begin. However, if you are still experiencing a lack of flexibility in your chest, back, neck, shoulders, or arm, you may need to see a physical therapist. Most women regain full range of motion and mobility within twelve weeks after surgery. Your surgeon probably gave you some gentle exercises to do before and following surgery. The daily stretch can advance these postoperative stretches and improve your freedom of movement once you are healed and fully recovered.

---

ing. A warm-up raises your body temperature, making your muscles more pliable.

- Do each stretch in a controlled manner. Do not bounce! Hold the steady stretch for ten to thirty seconds or more until you feel release in the muscle. A release is a feeling of "letting go" in the muscle or a sense that there is less tension on the muscles. Repeat stretching exercises five to ten times.
- Breathing promotes muscle relaxation. Holding your breath or inhaling often evokes muscle tension rather than muscle lengthening.
- Do not use your spine to stretch the muscles of the limbs (e.g., bending to touch your toes).
- The more frequently you stretch, the easier the exercises get and the more flexible your body stays. If you have trouble doing all the stretches every day, do half of them one day and the other half the following days. This will ensure that you get all of the stretches done at least three times a week.

The following daily stretch regimen should be safe for everyone regardless of joint problems. This regimen also enhances performance for any exercise you choose. Sport-specific stretching may need to be added to achieve greater results in performance.

When muscles are tight and unable to be stretched, massage can promote muscle relaxation. A massage can release deep tension in muscles,

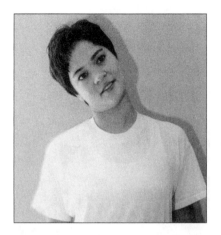

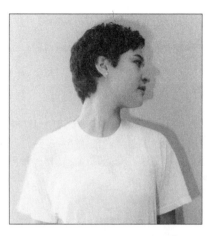

Neck stretch: Tilt. Tilt shoulder and hold ten seconds. Then slowly tilt head toward opposite shoulder and hold ten seconds. Repeat stretch five times on each side. Photos: Paul Zakar. Model: Mari O'Neill.

Neck stretch: Look. Turn head slowly to look over your shoulder. Hold ten seconds. Then slowly turn to look over the other shoulder and hold ten seconds. Repeat stretch five times on each side.

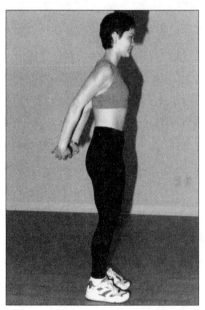

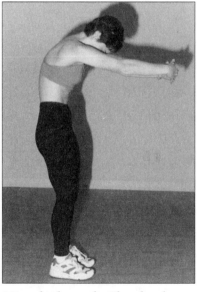

Chest stretch. Bring arms straight behind you as far as possible without pain. Hold ten seconds. Repeat five times, resting in between each stretch.

Upper back stretch. Clasp hands together in front with arms extended. Gently pull shoulder blades apart as you bend head comfortably forward. Hold for ten seconds. Repeat five times, resting in between each stretch.

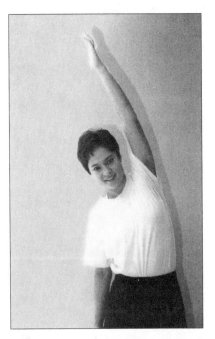 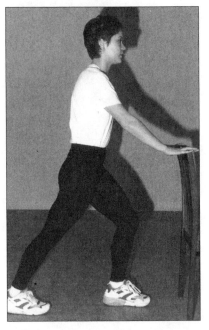

Side stretch. Stand with feet shoulder width apart and knees slightly bent. Bring arm up by ear. Keeping abdomen in, slowly bend to the side. Hold three seconds. Come back to center and slowly bend to the other side. Hold three seconds. Repeat stretch five times on each side. Photos: Paul Zakar. Model: Mari O'Neill.

Calf stretch. Keep back leg straight, with heel on the floor and toes pointed forward. Lunge toward the chair to feel stretch in back calf. Hold ten seconds. Repeat on each leg five to ten times.

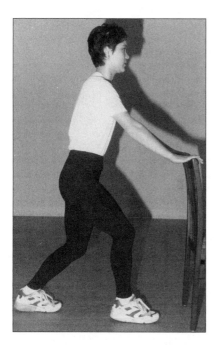

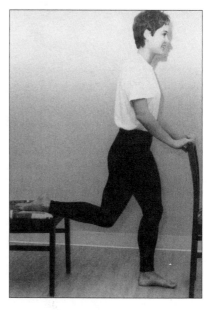

Soleus stretch. Keep back leg bent, with heel on the floor. Lean forward until you feel stretch in the lower calf area. Hold for ten seconds. Repeat five to ten times on each leg. Photos: Paul Zakar. Model: Mari O'Neill.

Quadriceps stretch. Support knee and lower leg on a chair as shown. Using the wall or another chair for balance, slowly bend standing leg until you feel stretch in the front of the thigh of the supported leg. Squeeze buttock of supported leg to increase stretch in the thigh and hip flexor muscles. Hold stretch for ten to twenty seconds and repeat five to ten times on each leg.

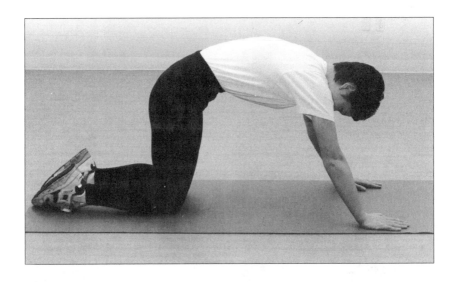

Cat stretch and camel relaxation. Begin on all fours with hands under shoulders and knees under hips in tabletop position: The tabletop position is a neutral position for the trunk. Your back is straight and your neck and head are in alignment with a straight back. Move into the cat stretch by pulling your abdominal muscles into your spine and tucking your pelvis under by arching up away from the floor. Your neck and head should follow and relax. Hold for five seconds, then slowly move into the camel relaxation position. Allow a gentle arch in your lower back and relax your belly. Head and chest are looking up without straining. Hold pose for five seconds. Repeat five times, alternating between the cat and camel. Photos: Paul Zakar. Model: Mari O'Neill.

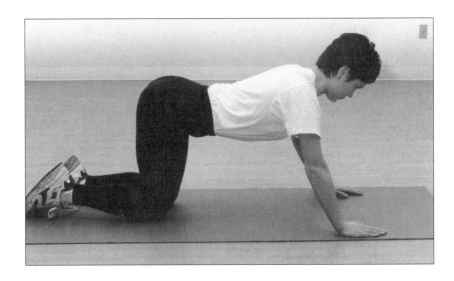

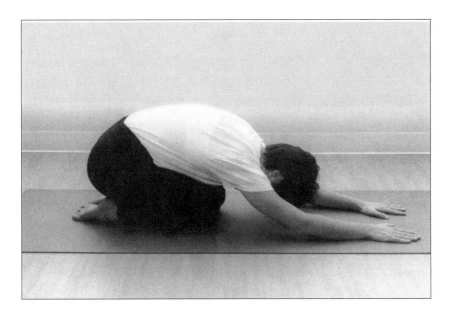

Child's pose. From an all-fours position, sit back onto the heels of the feet. Relax abdomen onto the legs/knees and upper body onto the floor to stretch the lower back. (A towel or pillow can be used behind the knee to decrease compression and strain on the knees.) Hold for five to ten seconds. Repeat five times, resting in between. Photos: Paul Zakar. Model: Mari O'Neill.

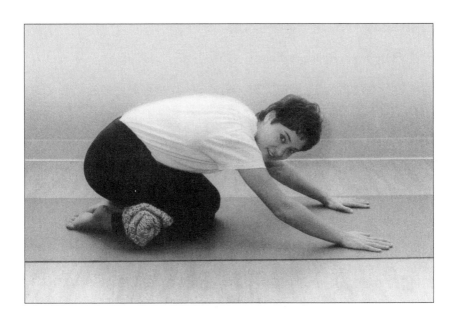

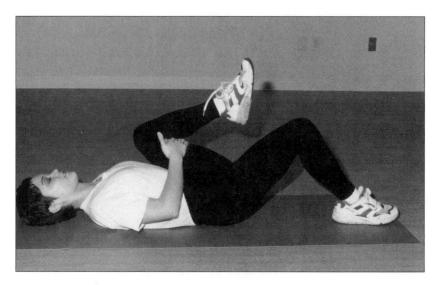

Knee to chest. Pull one knee into chest until you feel a comfortable stretch in the lower back and buttocks. Keep abdomen pulled in. Hold for five seconds and then slowly repeat with the other leg. Repeat five times on each side. Photos: Paul Zakar. Model: Mari O'Neill.

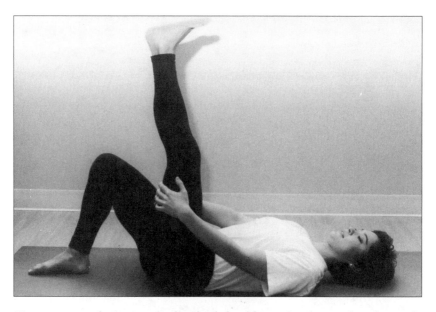

Hamstring stretch. Support back of leg behind knee. Gently straighten leg until you feel a comfortable stretch down the back of the leg. Hold stretch for ten to twenty seconds. Repeat five to ten times on each leg.

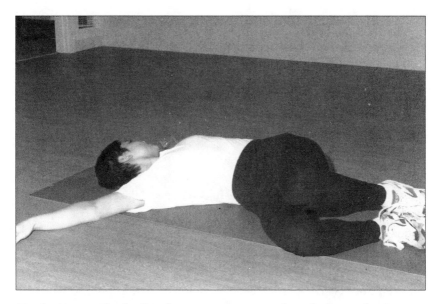

Trunk rotation. Slowly allow knees to rock to one side and relax on the floor. Hold for ten seconds or more. To change sides, pull in abdomen to support your back and slowly lift one leg at a time back to the starting position. Next, drop knees over to the opposite side. Repeat five times on each side. Pillow under head is optional. Photo: Paul Zakar. Model: Mari O'Neill.

freeing joints to move and be stretched. Massage allows your body time to let go of tension that may be causing pain or muscle dysfunction. Regular massage once or twice a month can prevent tension, pain, and injury. A licensed massage therapist charges about $50 per hour. You can find massage therapists at health clubs, in medical offices, and in private practice. Massage is now covered under some insurance plans. Ask your chiropractor or doctor for a recommendation for a massage therapist.

Tip for Breast Cancer Patients and Survivors

.⚘ There is some controversy about whether massage could spread cancer cells. However, many physicians believe that the benefits of massage for cancer patents far outweigh any potential risk. Be sure to check with your surgeon or oncologist before beginning therapeutic massage, however.

✍   The Pelvic Floor: The Forgotten Muscle

Exercise can be stressful for women who cannot be too far from a bathroom. Many women avoid exercising because they leak urine with movement due to weakened muscles that support their bladder. Activities such as jogging, high-impact aerobic classes, basketball, or just standing up or sneezing cause an increase in intra-abdominal pressure downward on the bladder and pelvic floor. This involuntary leakage with physical exertion is called urinary stress incontinence.

Some incontinent women can tolerate road biking but have problems with mountain biking because of the ups, downs, and bumps. Other women can walk flat surfaces but cannot tolerate the jarring of hiking or running, or horseback riding. Some women runners don't leak when running at a moderate pace but do leak when running at race pace or during sprints. The pelvic floor muscles act like a hammock that supports the internal organs, including the uterus. Pelvic floor muscles may be weaker for a woman who experienced an extreme amount of pushing, bearing down, or surgery during childbirth. According to the National Association for Incontinence, 46 percent of all incontinence in women is attributed to childbirth.

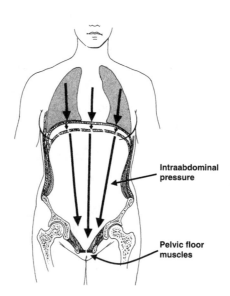

Intraabdominal
pressure

Pelvic floor
muscles

Figure 19.1. Stress incontinence. Reprinted by permission of Progressive Therapeutics, PC, 1998.

Estrogen helps to keep the urinary tract healthy. If you have low estrogen, as do postmenopausal women, you may be more prone to stress incontinence. Incontinence is not a problem only for older women, however. Some young women who have never had children can leak when they exercise. Several factors can irritate the bladder or pelvic muscles and make incontinence worse, including chronic constipation, weight gain, coffee, alcohol, citrus, milk products, smoking, and inactivity. As with any other muscle group, pelvic floor muscles become weak when they are not used. The good news is that weak pelvic floor muscles, like most other muscles, can be rehabilitated so that incontinence can be controlled.

In 1990, Dr. Ingrid Nyygard, a urogynecologist at the University of Iowa, conducted a study of 326 women with an average age of 38.5 years. Out of the 290 who reported regular exercise, 50 percent noted some incidence of incontinence. When asked how they handled the problem, 20 percent responded that they had stopped exercising, 18 percent had changed their exercise choice, and 55 percent continued to exercise but wore a pad for protection.

Exercises to increase pelvic floor tone and help alleviate incontinence were first developed more than fifty years ago by gynecologist named Arnold Kegel. The Kegel exercises we now recommend are to contract the muscles as if you were to stop the flow of urine, hold for ten seconds, rest for ten seconds, and repeat until gradually reaching 100 repetitions a day. Women may be able to clear up mild leakage problems with as few as twenty repetitions a day. The Kegel exercises can be done standing, lying down, or sitting. The best results are obtained when the exercise is repeated throughout the day. Be sure to

---

Tip for Breast Cancer Patients and Survivors

.✐ If you have experienced menopause due to cancer treatment and surgery, your estrogen levels are low and you may be more susceptible to incontinence. Even when the pelvic floor muscles are strong, the lack of estrogen may cause women to leak. If leaking is a constant and debilitating problem in your life, you should talk to your oncologist and gynecologist about treatment options.

keep your abdominal, buttocks, and inner leg muscles relaxed as you do Kegel exercise. Otherwise you reduce your ability to contract the pelvic floor muscles completely and cause an increase in pressure on the pelvic floor.

To avoid leakage during high-impact activities like running, it is important to learn to integrate the pelvic floor muscles into your workout. This means training the muscles to contract during peak tension moments, for example on impact of the ball, while stepping up or down on the curb when walking, or during jumps in your dance class. You can try strengthening your pelvic floor with a interval workout on a stair-climbing machine. Try holding the pelvic floor muscles contracted for a count of ten, then relax for ten seconds and repeat for a total of ten sets. Learning to isolate and then contract pelvic floor muscles during abdominal exercise or weight lifting further increases muscle control and strength. Usually, once a woman can locate and then properly contract the pelvic floor muscles her symptoms begin to improve immediately. Sometimes additional therapies, such as biofeedback, vaginal weights, or electrical muscle stimulation, are required to remedy symptoms of incontinence. For some women, medication or surgery may be needed. If you are having problems with incontinence, be sure to discuss them with your doctor.

Lower-Body Conditioning

There are three of choices for lower-body conditioning: cardiovascular or aerobic exercise, weight training, and isolated floor exercise. Weight-training machines when used correctly are a great option for improving the tone in the leg muscles and stability of the ankle, knee, and hip joints. Leg lifts and other floor exercises using ankle weights isolate and tone leg muscles, particularly the buttocks muscles, as effectively as or better than weight-training machines. Exercising with free weights and ankle weights isolates and firms the hip and buttocks muscles.

Strength in the buttocks area is important for the stability and support of the lower back. Aerobic exercise can improve the buttocks or leg muscles, resulting in more muscle isolation, toning, and support.

Stair-Climbing Machines

When exercising on a stair-climbing machine, pay attention to your form. Leaning forward too much reduces the amount of hip and buttocks muscles involvement and irritates your knees. The more involved you can make the hip and buttocks muscles, the more tone you gain in those muscle groups. Be sure to stand tall and press down through the heel of your foot, not the ball of your foot or toes. As you press down with the heel, be sure to intentionally contract the buttocks muscles. Your entire backside can get a great workout by just adjusting your form and focusing on using those muscles.

Bicycling (Indoors or Outdoors)

There is a misconception that cycling builds up your thigh muscles instead of reducing them. If you keep a high resistance on your bike all the time, you will increase the size of your muscles. However, if you maintain a higher cadence (the number of times the wheels revolve), you will find that cycling is an excellent way to strengthen leg muscles while trimming body fat. If the gears are set high, it will be difficult to turn the pedals and you have a lower cadence. It is better to decide how many rpm best suit your goals. If toning and trimming down the legs is your goal, you should spin your wheels at 90–100 rpm. If increasing muscle is your goal, keep your wheels spinning at 70 rpm or lower. Be careful not to strain your knee joints in the high gears and at low rpm. To find your cadence on a indoor bike, simply count revolutions of the front wheel for sixty seconds. For outdoor bikes, you can purchase an inexpensive device that straps to the tire and transmits a reading of rpm to a clock on your handlebars. If you can stand while biking, you increase the workout for your buttocks muscles.

Running, Walking, and Hiking

Walking and running lengthen and tone up leg muscles very quickly. There is no better way than walking or running to improve leg tone or overall lower-body condition. However, by analyzing your walking or running form you can become more efficient and faster and can reduce the chance of injury. Physical therapists do "gait analysis" in which they look at how you walk and teach you ways of walking to reduce injury and improve efficiency. How you run can also influence performance and injury risk. A running coach or trainer is a good resource for an analysis of your running stride. Including hills, intervals (speed workouts), and training drills in your regular walking or running program will help keep you interested and improve lower-body strength. Hiking places greater demands on the buttocks and hips due to the constant uphill and downhill motion.

In-Line Skating and Ice Skating

In-line skating is fun and provides a great workout for the legs and buttocks. In-line skating uses the inside and outside leg and buttocks muscles. The best time to contract the buttocks muscles is as you push off into a glide. After you push, make the pushing leg follow through on the motion and extend back. This increases the overall work of the back of

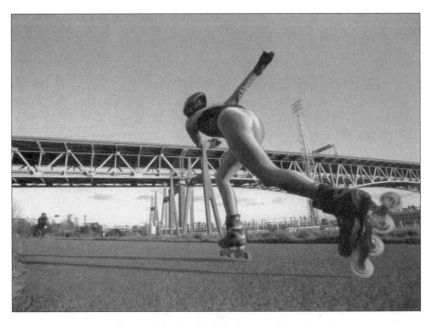

To increase the overall use of the back of the legs and buttocks, be sure to tighten the buttocks muscles as you extend the leg behind during the pushoff. Photo: Courtesy of K2 Corporation.

the legs and buttocks area. Be sure to ask your skate retailer for more information on skating form. In-line skating clubs are also good resources for improving form.

Squash, Tennis, and Other Racquet Sports

Racquet sports provide excellent exercise for leg tone because of the required running and sprinting. The lunging in these sports is a good workout for the buttocks muscles. Your inner and outer thigh muscles also get an excellent workout.

Horseback Riding

Horseback riding is an excellent exercise for increasing tone in the inner thighs. Depending on the style of riding and the amount of maintenance you personally do for the horse, caring for and riding a horse can be quite aerobic. When training, pay attention to your form and which muscles you are using to stabilize yourself. While riding, women find they get more use of their buttocks, pelvic floor, and inner leg muscles if they focus on using these muscles to keep a close attachment to the horse. When pulling up on the reins, use the legs and buttocks to stabilize that movement to increase the demand your lower body.

Abdominal Connection: Redeveloping Abdominal Tone

Many things affect the appearance of the abdomen. Some things are under your control, while many are not. Pregnancy causes changes in the abdominal muscles that are out of your control. Following pregnancy and childbirth, women often find that their waistline is thicker or that they just don't have a flat stomach any longer. Also, maintaining a trim waistline becomes more difficult as you age.

Your posture affects the look of your waistline and is a factor that you can control. When you slouch, your belly bulges and your abdomen looks much thicker than it is. If you have a tendency to have an exaggerated arch in your lower back (lordosis), your belly muscles become loose. The

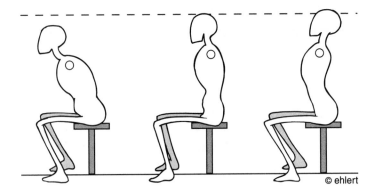

© ehlert

Figure 19.2. Good sitting posture improves abdominal tone.

posture that most affects the abdomen is prolonged sitting. Your abdomen does not work very much in a sitting position, and if you slouch when you sit, the weakening of the abdomen is even greater.

There are many ways to tone and strengthen the abdominal muscles, including high-tech machines and gimmicky exercise gear sold on TV. The quickest route to a flatter and more toned abdomen is the abdominal exercise you can do on the floor or bed. There are a variety of abdominal exercises that tone the abdomen. The partial sit-up known as the crunch is a good way to improve abdominal muscle strength. Daily abdominal exercise, however, is not enough to develop a flatter stomach. You need to learn to use the deep layers of the abdominal muscles in all of your activities in order to develop toned abdominal muscles. If you have back problems, crunches may be dangerous for you. The movement involved when performing a crunch may cause the vertebrae to rub together and irritate your spine. Be sure to check with your doctor before beginning abdominal exercise.

The technique for effective abdominal exercise begins with understanding the anatomy of the abdomen. The top layer of muscle is called the *rectus abdominis* and is primarily used for flexing the trunk. These muscles run vertically and are known by some as the "washboard" muscles. Below the rectus muscles, on either side of the abdomen are the *internal and external obliques.* The obliques bend and twist the torso. The deepest layer of muscle is the *transversus abdominis.* Because the job of the transversus abdominis is to pull the abdomen in, it is also the muscle that will flatten the abdomen the most. The transverse muscle is often weak and uninvolved. To contract the transverse muscle during abdominal exercise requires some thinking. Furthermore, the transverse muscle has a harder time contracting if it has become deconditioned from prolonged sitting.

Using the transverse muscle during exercise deepens the strength of the abdomen and gives more stability to the back. One reason the back may hurt during abdominal exercise is that the back muscles are inflexible; tight back muscles will be strained every time the trunk bends up into the crunch position. Learning to contract and then use the transverse muscles takes practice. If the transversus abdominis is weak, it is difficult to do contractions of the deep muscles, so the neck or back muscles will be substituted. It is important to train the transversus muscles with a variety of isometric exercises such as the transverse abdominis drill before trying to activate them during a crunch or other exercise. To integrate the transverse muscle into the crunch, you must learn to contract the deep muscle prior to lifting up into your crunch. This requires some coordination, but with practice and daily drills, you will develop an effective crunch. Another example of integrated abdominal use is during tennis. As you use your arm to hit the ball, tighten your abdominal muscles. This will not only increase the use of your abdomen during your tennis match but may also improve your game by putting more power behind the ball.

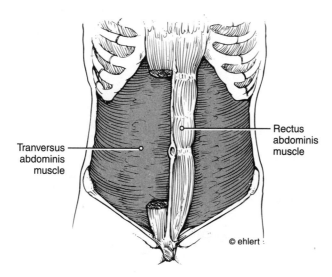

Figure 19.3. Abdominal muscles

Transverse Abdominal Drill

The transverse abdominal drill is a "sucking in" of the stomach to contract the deep muscles. While lying on the floor or bed, pull the abdomen in to the spine, keeping the natural curve in the lower back. Do not use the hips or legs to push the back into the floor. Next, keep the abdomen pulled in tight and pull the muscles in even more, bringing the spine toward the floor. This is an isolated contraction of the transverse muscles. Hold the contraction for ten seconds. Repeat ten times. Doing five to ten sets of ten repetitions a day will keep the deep muscles of the abdomen active. This drill can also be done in a sitting position or standing. The transverse muscles assist in exhalation; therefore, breathe out as the muscles contract inward.

Women who have had numerous surgeries in their back, chest, abdomen, and pelvic areas may need to do a fair amount of flexibility exercise along with their abdominal exercises to allow their muscles to contract freely. If your muscles are tight or restricted from scar tissue,

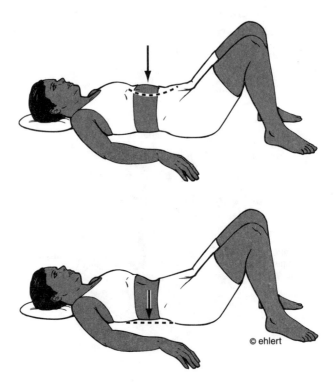

Figure 19.4. Transverse abdominal drill

Tip for Breast Cancer Patients and Survivors

The transverse abdominal drill is perfectly safe for breast cancer survivors who have had a mastectomy or reconstructive surgeries including the TRAM-flap (Transverse Rectus Abdominis Myocutaneous flap). Women feel the areas around their midsection, pelvis, and back become more unstable following the TRAM-flap surgery, and they are advised not to do abdominal exercises such as sit-ups or crunches to avoid hernia or other complications. However, during the TRAM-flap reconstruction, the transverse abdominal muscles are left intact and therefore can be strengthened safely using the transverse abdominal drill. This is an important muscle group to focus on postsurgery as long as you don't "bear down" and press outward with the belly muscles. Be sure to exhale while pulling the abdomen inward, bringing your belly button back toward your spine. As you hold the contraction in the abdomen, continue to breathe through the rib cage and chest area. If you have developed back pain or other discomforts following your surgeries, talk to your surgeon about abdominal exercise. Increasing the strength of the transverse muscles will increase low-back support. It is important that the exercise is done gently immediately following surgery, but as soon as possible after surgery is best.

---

just doing the simple transverse drill may be uncomfortable or painful. Gentle massage can help loosen up restricted muscles and improve your muscles' ability to contract fully and without pain.

The few minutes you spend doing abdominal exercise every day is not enough to keep tone in the abdomen. The key to maintaining abdominal tone is to use the abdominal muscles during daily activity and exercise. Weight-bearing exercise such as stair climbing or walking requires use of the abdomen for posture and balance. Non-weight-bearing exercise such as cycling or swimming does not naturally maximize the use of the abdominal muscles. You can get a great abdominal workout while swimming and biking if you concentrate on the abdomen and integrate the abdominal muscles into your form. If you can successfully integrate the use of the abdomen with exercise, you will also be able to use the abdominal muscles during physical activities such as gardening, lifting, or household chores.

Don't save abdominal exercise for the end of your workout where it may get left out. Do abdominal exercise after warm-up or stretching before you start your workout at the gym or go out for your walk. Making time to do an abdominal regimen is the first step in redeveloping a toned midsection. Integrating the deep muscles into your workout guarantees results.

Summary

- Conditioning exercise strengthens your muscles and joints and can improve performance with other exercises.
- Meditation and deep breathing can relax tense muscles, helping to reduce pain and chance of injury.
- Stretching is extremely important to prevent muscle and tendon injury.
- Many women are prone to incontinence, mostly due to weak pelvic floor muscles. These muscles can be strengthened with special exercises, which reduce urinary leakage.
- Lower-body conditioning can be done with a combination of weight-training machines and free weights. Some aerobic exercise, such as walking, hiking, biking, and in-line skating, also provides excellent lower-body conditioning.
- Abdominal muscle conditioning exercises can improve the appearance of your abdomen while helping to strengthen and stabilize back muscles.

20

Exercise Choices

Are you wondering what type of exercise is best or what exercise plan is going to give you the most return on your time investment? The answer is whatever exercise you like and will actually do. In order to succeed in exercise, you need to like what you do and the exercise needs to fit into your lifestyle. In this chapter we describe several ways of exercising, including exercising on your own, exercising with a fitness buddy, and joining a team sport. We outline several specific activities that might interest you. We then describe the several different modes of exercising, including home activities, fitness centers or gyms, and sports.

We are fortunate to have so many more exercise choices than women had fifty years ago. You may have noticed more exercise choices available in the past year compared to previous years. As the fitness market continues to grow and add new exercise options, some women feel that they have too many exercise choices.

Specific goals require specific exercise action plans. However, before you can decide when and how long you will exercise, you need to find the type of exercise that best fits your lifestyle. For optimal results, the exercise you choose must be done consistently, so you must like what you are doing. It may take some time to discover what kind of physical activity touches your soul and keeps you coming back for more.

First, decide what kind of person you are and how you like to spend your time. If you like solitary time, exercising on your own may work for you. If you need to have a close friend or buddy with you to make an activity enjoyable, you might opt for partnered sports. If you like to do things as part of a group, you might fit in well with a team sport. Many women find that they enjoy doing a variety of all three types of activities.

Exercising on Your Own

Many women have such busy schedules that adding another class or meeting doesn't work for them. They have to fit in exercise when they can, and it may be at a different time each day. For such women, exercising on their own may work best. Or you might value having some solitary time, especially if you otherwise have a day full of meetings, kids, errands, etc. Biking, weight lifting, in-line skating, running, and walking are exercises that you can do on your own and do not require a partner, instructor, or group.

Walking

Walking is an excellent exercise that you can do on your own with very little investment in equipment. A good pair of supportive walking shoes

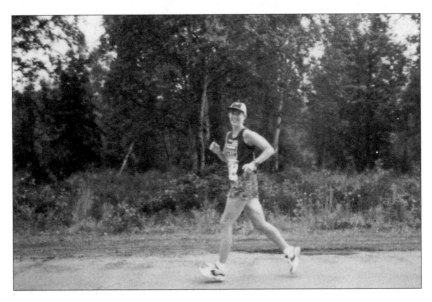

Running does not require a partner, instructor, or group.

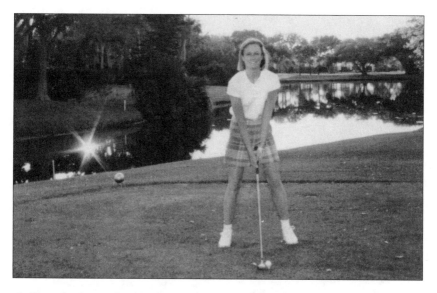

Golf can be done solo or with a partner or group and is fun, low-level aerobic exercise.

is all that is required. At a low to moderate intensity, walking can help to manage body weight. Walking also encourages your bones to increase in strength, which is important for preventing osteoporosis. Walking can be your main source of exercise or it can complement a non-weight-bearing aerobic regimen such as riding a stationary bike or swimming.

The best way to start a walking program is to set a goal. You may want to walk five days a week, compete in a marathon, or walk your daily three-mile loop in less than an hour. For models on how to identify a goal and plan your progressive walking program, see the sample progressive walking programs in Chapter 14.

Partnered Exercise or Clubs

Walking on your own is convenient; you don't have to schedule with any-one or keep to someone else's exercise plan. However, if you are having difficulty walking on your own, or you would just like some social sup-port, walking is easy to do with other people and provides social time with friends or coworkers. Another option is to join a walking group. Walking groups or clubs meet for weekly walking sessions and may also

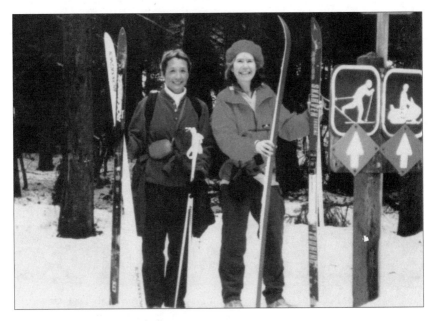

Cross-country skiing is excellent aerobic exercise and safer with a partner. Photo: Lisa Talbott.

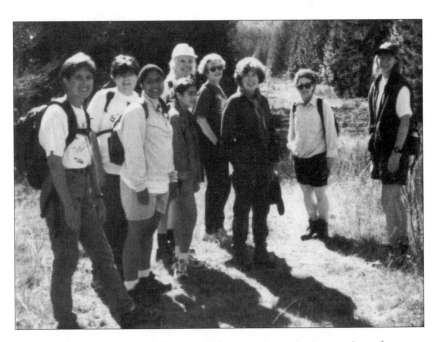

Walking and hiking with a group or club gives you a core group of people to exercise with and help keep you motivated. Photo: Lisa Talbott.

participate in local walking events. Local walking events can help you to set goals to work toward. A club, such as a cycling or running club, gives you a core group of people to train with and provides social support, which can be very motivating and makes exercise fun. The weekly sessions also create a scheduled time to exercise. When you have an exercise session scheduled with someone or with a group, you are less likely to miss that session. Racquet sports such as tennis and racquetball are other partnered sports.

Team sports are another way to obtain support for exercising. Many women never had the opportunity in high school or college to play team sports. Fortunately, there now are community teams that are noncompetitive for women of all ages. It is common to find "over 40" sport teams that do not require any previous experience. Soccer, basketball, rowing, and swimming are all effective aerobic exercise that can offer fun with women your own age. These sports help you stick to your fitness plan because they require practices and games that work like any other scheduled workout time. Some sports, such as softball and volleyball, are not as aerobic as others, but they too have scheduled practices. They are also good for building overall body strength. If your goal is to reduce fat and increase aerobic exercise, a sport such as volleyball

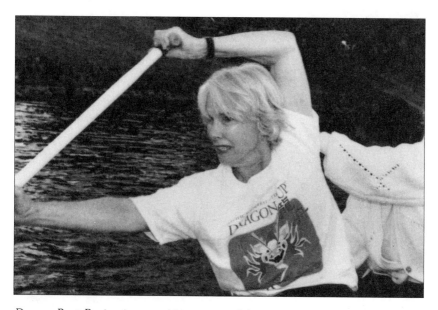

Dragon Boat Racing is an exciting team activity.

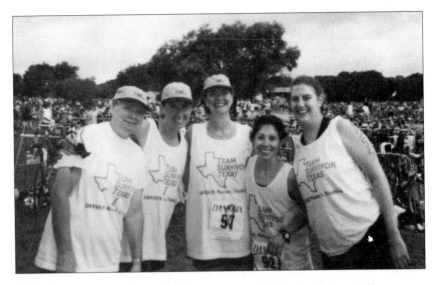

Texas Team Survivor (left to right) Marcia McClellan, coach Lisa Talbott, Karen Boatright, Shirley Sanchez, coach Laurie Rourke

or softball would be better suited as a complement to another form of aerobic exercise.

Racquet Sports

Tennis, squash, and other racquet sports can build both aerobic ability and strength. Racquet sports require a partner, so you'll have a workout buddy with you to keep you motivated. Although these sports can be played noncompetitively, there is still an element of self-competition. Healthy self-competition is an excellent motivator. Although winning may be what motivates you, challenging yourself to play better and improve your skill could be even more intriguing than winning.

Fitness Centers

Many team sports and clubs are found in the community or at fitness centers. Fitness centers offer a variety of exercise opportunities. Here are a few options.

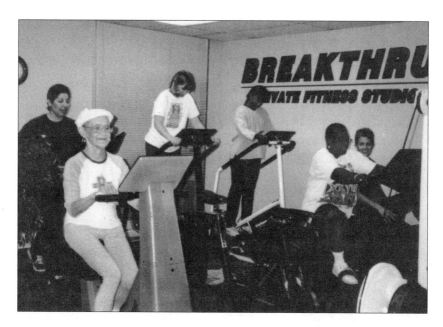

Fitness centers offer a variety of exercise options. Photo: Karen Van Kirk.

Health Clubs

Health clubs come in all sizes and shapes. The differences among health clubs are the types of services they provide. Gyms that offer limited exercise opportunities are less expensive than the more full-service luxury health clubs. A gym that offers only weight training and aerobic equipment maybe cost you as little as $20 a month. The locker rooms in this type of gym will also be very basic and you will need to bring your own towel and lock. Clubs that offer classes such as aerobics and yoga, quality trainers, or baby-sitting may cost $50 per month or more. This type of facility may also provide towels and free orientation sessions with a qualified trainer to get you started.

As more services are offered, the price of the health club goes up. If the club offers swimming, tennis, and other facilities such as a basketball or squash courts, the cost may be well over $100 per month. The bigger, more luxurious health clubs often offer social events and may organize seasonal opportunities such as a downhill ski club. These facilities may also have a spa, dry cleaning service, or a travel agent on site.

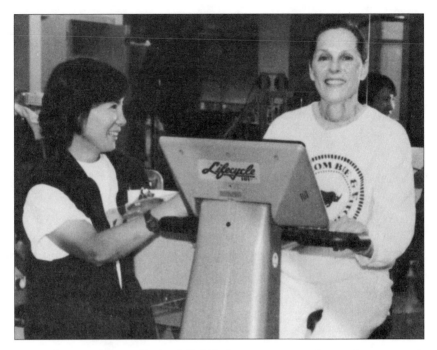

Personal trainer Monica Packard (left) helps women set and meet their personal goals.

Personal Training Facilities

Personal training facilities are gyms that provide basic equipment, but you are required to hire one of their trainers. Personal training facilities can be your primary source of exercise, or you can visit just once a month to update your program.

Specialty Clubs

Some fitness centers are designed to attract a certain type of person or group. For example, a club may buy equipment that best suits certain team sports or offer classes that attract seniors, such as water aerobics. The best examples are the all-women clubs. These facilities are designed with women in mind, so they focus on exercise opportunities that will attract women, such as weight-lifting equipment made specifically for women. There are clubs that focus on exercise classes that attract both women and men. Fitness classes can range from a variety of aerobics classes to weight-lifting and strength-building classes or complementary classes such as abdominal conditioning or yoga. Some facilities offer only exercise classes and may be called "aerobics studios." The popular cycling or spinning classes done on stationary bikes are often found in a dedicated studio. Many dance studios have now expanded beyond traditional dance for children and are offering adult dance classes and other forms of movement such as tai chi, yoga, or swing dance.

Community Centers, Wellness Centers, and Senior Centers

Community, wellness, and senior centers offer activities for a variety of groups. Community centers tend to be family-oriented, offering exercise classes for people of all ages. Wellness centers may offer classes for special populations such as cancer or arthritis patients. These facilities are designed to accommodate these individuals' physical needs and they offer other services that increase patients' quality of life. Senior centers offer exercise classes specifically designed for seniors. Some include

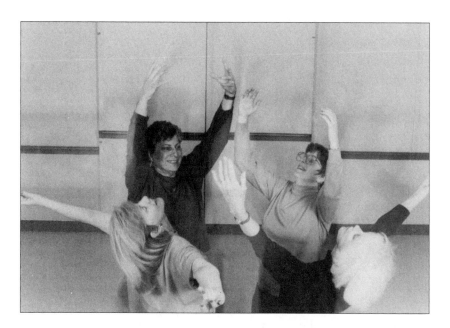

Dance, movement, and exercise classes for all ages can be found at fitness centers, specialty clubs, and community centers.

wellness programs with lectures on managing arthritis, incontinence, or other problems. Some also offer nutrition and cooking classes.

Home Exercise

Although there are many places you can go to exercise, you may prefer exercising at home. This can range from going for a walk or bike ride from home to setting up a home "gym" environment that encourages exercise. It is best if you have space where exercise equipment can stay and not have to be moved every time you want to work out. If you have an extra room and can dedicate the space for exercise, you will have the most success because you will be less distracted by other things around the house you need to do. Placing your equipment in front of a TV or window with a view helps make the exercise time go by faster. Before you spend a lot of money on home equipment, however, make sure that it will work for you. One of the more common uses of home exercise equipment is to hang laundry on! If a friend of yours has home equipment, you might ask to use hers a couple of times, to determine if this is something you would enjoy and stick with. Many health clubs offer a one-day "guest" membership for a small fee, so you can check out all the equipment. Avoid gimmicky devices—it's best to stick with simple models of equipment. If you can afford it, an electronic treadmill gives the highest intensity home workout. If you want something more economical, you can find inexpensive stationary bikes. Hand weights, as we mentioned in Chapter 18, are very inexpensive.

If you do not have space for equipment, you can buy or rent exercise videos. There are hundreds of videos that range from aerobics to yoga. You can also check out videos from your local public library.

To be successful exercising at home you must be strategic, regardless of the mode of exercise you choose. Do your exercise program when you can give it your full attention: turn the ringer on your phone off, turn down the volume on your answering machine, turn off your pager and cell phone. Tell your family or housemates not to interrupt you for the period of time you need to finish your program. The most common mistake women make when exercising at home is to start and stop and never complete their workout. They pedal on the bike for ten minutes and then remember a call they had to make and get off the bike. Fifteen minutes later they get back on for five minutes and then decide they really need to go move the laundry. Then they come back in twenty minutes and get back on the bike or get distracted and never get back on the bike and finish the session. Don't let your exercise session drag out like this; it will wear you out and make exercising a chore.

Many women exercise in their office. If you are fortunate to have a large enough space at work to set up an office gym, this may be a good option for you. Exercising during lunchtime or after a long meeting is convenient and gives you a healthy way to take breaks and maintain your energy.

Outdoor Wilderness and Adventure Sports

Many women are choosing to brave the elements and enjoy the exhilaration of doing an outdoor wilderness sport. These can range from nature walks and hikes to mountain climbing. Depending on where you live, you can find organizations that lead certain types of expeditions. They usually include training classes so that you can be well prepared before you start your adventure. Here in the Pacific Northwest we have many outdoor sports from which to choose, such as sea kayaking, rock climbing, ice

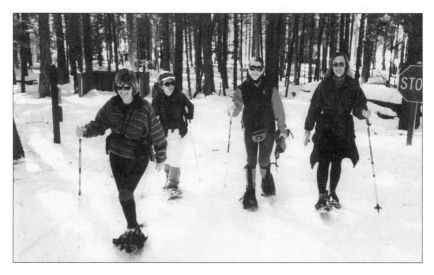

Snowshoeing is just like hiking or walking trails except that you are on snow!
Photo: Lisa Talbott.

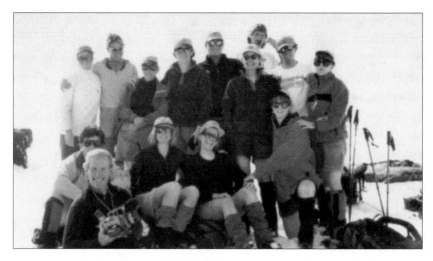

Team Survivor Northwest at Camp Miur on top of 14,400-foot Mt. Rainier

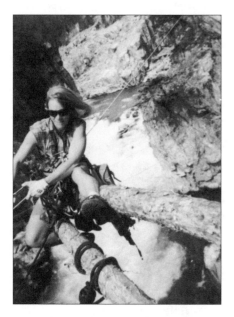

Jazz Scheingraber is an all-around athlete who uses a variety of exercises and sport to stay fit. Cross-country skiing, adventure and triathlon racing, and rock climbing are just a few of the activities that Jazz enjoys doing and coaching.

climbing, mountain climbing (Mount Rainier is a favorite of the locals), and mountain biking. More traditional outdoor sports are available around the country, including crosscountry and downhill skiing, swimming, canoeing, and rowing. Needless to say, these sports are best done with a partner or a group.

Using a Variety of Exercise

If you like variety in your exercise, try different modes. Walking, running, biking, swimming, and weight lifting are all cheap and accessible, and you can do them alone. Yoga and martial arts such as aikido build muscle strength and upper-body power. Although they are not aerobic, these forms of exercise help the body, mind, and spirit and are an excellent adjunct to your aerobic program. Changing your exercise plan every few months to adapt to the seasons is a healthy way to stay active year-round. Allow yourself a variety of exercise to keep you motivated. You will be pleased with the results and will have fun along the way.

Summary

- To be effective and sustainable, exercise must be interesting.
- Women have many choices for exercise today.
- You can choose to exercise on your own, with a partner, on a team, in exercise classes, or in some combination of these.
- Walking is an excellent exercise that can be done on your own, with a partner, or as part of a group. It can be recreational or competitive.
- Racquet sports are excellent sports if you enjoy working out with a partner.
- There are many team sports options available for women today, even for those who have never done sports before.
- Many women enjoy working out in a fitness facility. There are many different types from which to choose.
- You can make your home into a "gym" by purchasing some home equipment such as a stationary bicycle or hand weights.
- Many women are opting for outdoor wilderness sports.

21

Fitting Exercise
into a Busy Life

The most common reason we hear from women who do not exercise is, "I don't have the time to exercise." A regular exercise program needs to be scheduled into your week just like hair appointments and business lunches. This is not about having the time, but about making the time. In this chapter we give you several tips on how you can make exercise a routine part of your life.

Schedule It in and Monitor Your Progress

Start by writing your workouts into your day timer or calendar for the first month. This helps to establish when exercise fits in best to your current schedule. For some women, exercise fits in best before or after work. For others, it's a daily decision as they book other appointments or have rotating work schedules. The key is to write down your workout plan and make it a priority. The goal is to learn to schedule your life around your workout sessions rather than fitting exercise around your life. There is *always* something else to be doing, something else that feels more important. Until you start making yourself and your exercise plan the most important part of your day, you will continually be fighting an uphill battle to find the time you deserve for yourself.

You can use some other tools for monitoring your progress. One tool to help you keep track of how much walking you do is a pedometer. This is an inexpensive little monitor you wear on your pants or skirt at the waist that counts up your steps. One mile equals about 1,740 steps. Most women walk about two to three miles a day just doing their daily routines. Researchers have found that people who walk 10,000 or more steps a day have significant improvements in weight, insulin, and other health factors. If you walk three miles a day for exercise and do three miles in your daily routine, you'll easily be over the 10,000-step mark.

Exercise in the Morning

If anytime is good for you to exercise, do it in the morning. Morning exercise starts your day with a healthy attitude, gets your workout out of the way, and leaves less chance of it being left off your list of "things to do today." Some research suggests that exercise done first thing in the morning may have the most benefit on weight control, insulin, and growth factors that can be important in cancer prevention. We have also found that clients and patients who change to morning workouts find it easier to stay on their eating plans.

Make Exercise a Routine Part of Your Day

Some of our patients and clients feel they have met their fitness goals when they have lost the ten pounds they wanted to lose. We believe that they have reached their goal when exercise is part of their day, like brushing their teeth. You don't schedule brushing your teeth and you don't think about it—you just do it because it is a habit you learned when you were a child and you know it is the best way to prevent dental health problems. Why would daily exercise, which helps keep your whole body healthy, be any different? Figure out what is getting in the way of your workouts and you will be one step closer to a regular exercise program— and a body you are proud of. When logging your workouts the first month, pay attention to why you didn't work out when you had scheduled exercise time. If it is a special project for work that always keeps you late at the office, do that project first in the morning, set a specific time to stop working on it, and leave time to exercise. Does your job as taxi driver for your kids interfere with a regular exercise plan? Try going for a walk or

Tip for Breast Cancer Patients and Survivors

✐ The added time commitments of doctors' appointments, chemotherapy, and support groups can add a burden to your hectic life. Getting help is the best way to allow yourself time for taking care of yourself, including exercising. If you can, think about taking a leave of absence from work or cut down on your work hours for a few months. Make sure that you get plenty of rest—you will need it for the increased demands of treatment on your body. Save your energy for a daily walk rather than cleaning the house if walking is something that you enjoy. Ask family and friends to help with child care, chores, and errands. People usually enjoy helping out.

run while waiting for your children to finish soccer practice. Better still, walk with another soccer mom during the practice. Ask for support from others and support yourself. Don't give up—look for more solutions. Everyone has challenges to maintaining a regular exercise program.

✐   Substitute

It is surprising how much time even the busiest women can find in their days. You just need to look for unnecessary things you do and replace them with exercise. You can easily cut out an hour of television each week and go for a walk instead. Or recycle those catalogs that arrive in the mail rather than poring over them. You can spend the extra half hour doing some weight training. If you love to read, do it while you are on a stationary bike. Instead of going to a bar to sit and drink with friends, convince them to join you for a night of dancing. Opt for a bike ride on a Saturday instead of a movie. There are undoubtedly many areas of your life where you could substitute an active activity for a sedentary one.

✐   Bring Exercise and Movement into
All Parts of Your Life

If you have a hard time getting all of your exercise program into your busy day, try fitting pieces of it in here and there throughout the day. Research has shown that doing several short bouts of exercise has the same benefit on weight control as doing one longer stretch of exercise. The important thing is that you keep track of what you are doing. As we describe in Chapter 16, you can exchange higher-energy activities for sedentary activities.

- Opt for stairs rather than an elevator for fewer than five floors. Waiting for an elevator, and waiting while it opens and closes on several floors, takes time. You can often take the stairs in the same or less time than using the elevator. Doctors and other emergency hospital staff have known this for a long time. Where there is an emergency code in the hospital everyone heads for the stairs because it's faster than waiting for an elevator. Taking stairs up to the next floor uses about twenty calories for a woman who weighs about 150 pounds. If you take stairs five times a day, you've burned an extra 100 calories!

- When you are sitting at your computer, move your legs. Shake them up and down. Get a stationary cycle. Or use a vertically adjustable table for your computer so that you have the option of not sitting down all day long.

- Walk over to your coworker rather than sending an E-mail.

- Make lunchtime walking appointments with colleagues and friends instead of high-calorie lunch dates.

- Make and keep exercise "dates" with your friends or family. Take a bike ride together instead of driving to a fast-food restaurant to meet for lunch.

- Take a ten-minute exercise break at work. Stretch, take a quick walk. You will feel much more energized for the next few hours.

- If you have a choice, live within walking or biking distance of your work.

- Go dancing with your spouse instead of to the movies. Avoid alcohol when you go dancing—it includes empty calories, makes you dehydrated, and decreases your coordination, making you more prone to injury.

- Take active destination vacations rather than driving trips. Many resorts have a variety of activities and sports. If you want a low-key option, go to a resort that has bike and walking trails, swimming pools, etc. If you are more adventurous, look for outdoor adventure trips.

- Avoid drive-through restaurants and stores. Stop your car, get out, and walk into the store or restaurant. Most drive-through restaurants do not have many low-calorie, healthy food choices anyway.

- Don't stockpile things that need to go upstairs or to another room in your house to make the trip all at once. Make several trips a day up and down the stairs in your house. Wear a pedometer every day and watch your daily steps increase.

Summary

- Everyone can find time to add exercise to her daily life. The key is to *make* the time.
- You need to schedule exercise into your day so that other things do not take priority.
- Exercising in the morning gets it out of the way first thing and may have special health benefits.
- Make exercise a routine part of your day.
- Try different types of exercise to keep you interested.
- Walking is excellent exercise that can easily be added throughout the day.
- Choose high-energy over sedentary activities when you have a choice.

22

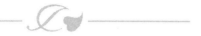

Exciting New Research in
Exercise and Breast Cancer

We have presented the results of several studies on the association between exercise and breast cancer and on the other health effects of exercise. There are still many open questions about the role of exercise in preventing new or recurrent breast cancer, however. To answer these open questions, Drs. Anne McTiernan and Julie Gralow and other researchers are conducting exciting new studies that will provide important information. Dr. McTiernan is a physician and epidemologist and studies the effect of exercise on breast cancer incidence and on some of the risk factors for breast cancer. Dr. Gralow is an oncologist specializing in breast cancer and is involved in several clinical trials in breast cancer treatment. We describe some of our new research endeavors on exercise and breast cancer in this chapter.

Exercise's Effect on Hormones in Postmenopausal Women

Dr. Anne McTiernan is principal investigator of the Physical Activity for Total Health study, which is a clinical trial testing the effect of two different exercise programs on blood estrogens and androgens (e.g., testosterone) in postmenopausal women. This study is being done at the Fred Hutchinson Cancer Research Center and is funded by the National Cancer Institute. We have recruited about 170 women who are healthy, sedentary, and not using hormone therapy, and whose percent body fat is 32 or greater. The women are enrolled into one of the two programs: an aerobic (walking and cycling) and weight-training program, and a stretching exercise program. Since it is a clinical trial, the women are placed at random into one of the two exercise programs. Each woman stays in her program for a year. During the year, we take many measurements, including exercise, fitness, height and weight, body-fat measures, blood measures, and diet, and we distribute questionnaires. At the end of the study, in approximately 2001, we will be able to say with certainty whether exercise can lower blood estrogen levels in postmenopausal, overweight women. We also hope to get funding to look at the effect of the exercise programs on some features of the women's mammograms to determine if exercise can reduce breast density, which is an important risk factor for breast cancer.

Exercise's Effect on Immune Function in Postmenopausal Women

In another study associated with Physical Activity for Total Health, Dr. McTiernan and her colleagues are looking at the effect of the exercise programs on immune function. As we described in Chapter 6, your body's immune system may be very important in fighting cancer. We suspect that exercise may be one tool to boost your immunity. This study will tell us if an aerobic or stretching exercise program benefits such immune system cancer fighters as natural killer cells, cytokines, or some antibodies.

Exercise and Breast Cancer Recurrence and Survival

Dr. McTiernan is also collaborating with Dr. Gralow and other investigators at the Fred Hutchinson Cancer Research Center, the University of Washington, the National Cancer Institute, the University of Southern California, and the University of New Mexico. We are studying a cohort of breast cancer patients to look at the effect of exercise, body fat, blood estrogens and other hormones, and other factors on breast cancer recurrence and survival. We are following about 1,200 patients, many of whom are African-American or Latina. That way, we will be able to look at exercise effects in a variety of breast cancer patients. This study is called the HEAL Study, which stands for Health, Eating, Activity, and Lifestyle.

✐ Exercise and Breast Cancer Risk in Postmenopausal and Older Women

Dr. McTiernan is an investigator with the Women's Health Initiative, which collects detailed information about current and past exercise habits. As a result, we will have the ability to describe the associations between exercise frequency and amount on several chronic diseases that affect postmenopausal and older women. We are now starting to look at the effect of exercise on breast cancer development in the WHI participants. We will have the unique ability to look at the exercise effects while controlling for measures of body weight, body fat distribution, and diet. Results from that analysis should be available sometime in the year 2000. In WHI, all participants are followed long-term, so in the future we will also be able to look at the effect of exercise on breast cancer survival.

✐ Exercise and Diet Effects in Breast Cancer Patients

A few years ago Dr. McTiernan, Dr. Gralow, and other colleagues published results of a pilot study of exercise and diet in breast cancer patients. We wanted to see if we could recruit breast cancer patients to a study that involves two major lifestyle changes—a low-fat diet and a thrice-weekly aerobic exercise program in an exercise facility. We found first of all that the patients were very interested in such a program. We sent invitation letters with enclosed questionnaires to 100 patients who had been referred to us by their physicians. More than forty patients were ready and willing to make some major changes in their lives, and they were willing to do so by contributing to a research study. When researchers recruit for participants in these sorts of studies, they usually find that fewer than 5 percent of people are willing to commit themselves to a research intervention study. Out of the forty interested patients, ten were eligible and were enrolled in the study. Nine completed the study and made substantial improvements in their fitness, diet, and body fat.

Exercise's Effects on Bone in Breast Cancer Patients

Dr. Anna Schwartz and Dr. Gralow have been funded to test the effects of exercise and the drug raloxifene on markers of bone strength in breast cancer patients. Young (premenopausal) breast cancer patients often stop having periods and become postmenopausal as a result of their chemotherapy treatment. The result of this early change in menstrual function is that they have very low levels of estrogen, which protects their breasts but which causes their bones to become weak and osteoporotic. This study, a controlled clinical trial, will provide answers about what breast cancer survivors can do to protect other aspects of their long-term health in addition to their breast health.

Summary

- The Physical Activity for Total Health study is measuring the effect of exercise on estrogen and other hormones in post-menopausal women.
- The Physical Activity for Total Health study is also assessing exercise effect on markers of immune function in older women.
- The Health, Eating, Activity, and Lifestyle study is following a group of breast cancer patients to look at the associations among physical activity, diet, weight, body fat, mammogram features, genetics, blood hormones, and breast cancer prognosis and quality of life.
- The Women's Health Initiative will contribute information on the effect of exercise on breast cancer in older women.
- Seattle researchers continue to study exercise effects on various markers of disease and health in breast cancer patients.

23

How You Can Help

We have talked with many women around the country about breast cancer. Many have asked us what they can do to join the fight against breast cancer. Some have had breast cancer recently, some in the remote past. Others have watched their mothers, sisters, daughters, friends, and other loved ones struggle with the disease. In this chapter we give you some ideas of ways you can contribute to the effort.

Fighting breast cancer is similar to fighting an enormous forest fire. The people fighting the fire would have no hope of controlling it if they attacked the fire with only one bucket brigade on one side of the fire. Firefighters usually attack a forest fire on several sides at one time, and sometimes even from the sky. Similarly, the fight against breast cancer needs to be fought on all of its fronts—cure, treatment, prevention, and early diagnosis. We need to find new and better treatments. We should test methods to help women better cope with living with breast cancer. We must discover better ways to detect breast cancer at an early stage, to increase the chances for a cure. We have to research prevention methods, so that in the future, breast cancer will once again be a rare disease that most of our daughters and granddaughters will not have to worry about.

The fight against breast cancer needs to be fought by all women. We as researchers and clinicians can do only so much. It is going to be the combined efforts of patients, women at risk, their families and friends, and professionals that wins the war. Breast cancer has claimed more

American lives since 1960 than did World War II and the Korean, Vietnam, and Gulf wars combined. The war against breast cancer is truly a world war that we must all fight together.

There are many ways that you can help in the fight against breast cancer. You have some particular gift that you can give to the cause.

Volunteer Your Time and Services

If you are retired, or have some free time, you can volunteer your time to a local breast cancer organization. If you have leadership experience, you can lend that to the organization. If your experience runs more to word processing or stuffing envelopes, then offer that kind of support. There are several national and local breast cancer activist organizations and research support organizations that could use your help. The Susan G. Komen Breast Cancer Foundation was founded in 1982 by Nancy Brinker, herself a breast cancer survivor, in honor of her sister, who died of breast cancer at age thirty-six. The Komen Foundation is dedicated to raising awareness of breast cancer and to supporting education, patient care, and research in breast cancer. The Komen Foundation's Race for the Cure occurs in dozens of U.S. cities each year to raise breast cancer awareness and funds to support research, outreach, and education projects. The American Cancer Society funds multiple studies on breast cancer prevention and treatment, and brings breast cancer programs to women all over the country. Team Survivor USA has chapters in many areas of the country, and new chapters are opening each year. There are many other local and national organizations that you can contact. We have listed some of the national organizations in Appendix B. You can find your local organizations by looking in the phone book under "cancer" or by calling your local hospital.

Join a Study

There are hundreds of studies of breast cancer risk and treatment that could use your help at one time or another. Less than 3 percent of cancer patients in this country are enrolled in clinical trials. And yet the cancer patients who are in trials have better survival than those who are not in these studies. We cannot learn about new ways to treat breast cancer if patients do not agree to test new promising therapies. Ask your doctor if there are any studies recruiting patients in your area in which you could participate.

The cost of participating is usually borne by the study, although you and your insurance company may be charged for tests and procedures that you would have had if you were not in a clinical trial. Many insurance companies will not pay for treatment that is part of a clinical trial. This policy may be changing. People who get their health insurance though the Department of Defense can enroll in National Cancer Institute–sponsored clinical trials, and the Department of Defense will cover the cost of the trials. Other insurance companies may soon follow suit.

If you have concerns about being in an "experiment" or worry that you would be a "guinea pig" if you joined a clinical trial, you can rest assured that there is a safety committee, usually called an Institutional Review Board, associated with the institution sponsoring the clinical trial. You can call the director of the Institutional Review Board if you have questions or concerns about a particular clinical trial. Any clinician or researcher in this country who wants to do a study involving humans as subjects has to have the research plan and procedures approved by one of these Institutional Review Boards. The Institutional Review Boards have to follow certain guidelines set down by the United States government to assure that there is no abuse, mistreatment, or dishonesty on the part of the researcher or institution, and that the safety of the study participants is assured to the highest degree possible. Furthermore, all clinicians and researchers are required to explain the study fully to you and carefully explain the potential risks and benefits of participating in the study.

If you do not have breast cancer, there are many studies in which your participation could be a real contribution. The Study of Tamoxifen and Raloxifene (STAR) trial is looking for postmenopausal women at increased risk for breast cancer to participate in a study comparing tamoxifen and raloxifene as drugs to reduce the risk of developing breast cancer. If you are called or asked to participate in a study as a "normal control," agree to answer the questions. Your participation could be critical to the results. Of course, you should determine that any invitation is legitimate. If you have any questions, ask the person recruiting you what research institution she or he is representing, and call that institution to make sure that the study is legitimate.

Ask Your Representatives and Senators to Support Breast Cancer Research

Most of the cancer research dollars in this country come from the National Cancer Institute. Congress funds the National Cancer Institute; each year, the overall government budget and the allocation that Congress gives to it determine its budget.

The National Cancer Institute is charged with sponsoring and doing research into the causes, prevention, and treatment of cancer. Most of the studies of exercise and breast cancer have been funded through the National Cancer Institute. The National Cancer Institute is also very well suited to look at the big picture of cancer research and to spend research dollars according to greatest need. The National Cancer Institute has developed an excellent system to get expert scientific input from around the country and around the world to advise on what they fund and what they do. There is no other government or private institute that can match their expertise. One thing that you can do is to ask your representative and senator to increase funding for breast cancer research through the National Cancer Institute. You can specifically ask that research on exercise and breast cancer be done. If enough women ask for this, Congress may make it a priority for the National Cancer Institute to include in their research agenda.

The Centers for Disease Control and Prevention does some cancer research and funds research around the country. The focus of this government institution, however, is different from that of the National Cancer Institute. The Centers for Disease Control and Prevention is involved more in surveillance and control of disease epidemics. This organization funds studies and programs to increase the access of poor women to mammogram screening, for example. If your special interest is in helping poor and underserved women to get access to good medical care, prevention, and treatment, you could ask your representatives to make sure that the Centers for Disease Control and Prevention has an adequate budget to accomplish its missions.

✍ Give Financial Support

Although the United States government funds millions of dollars in breast cancer research each year, it is never enough to find all of the answers soon enough. Cancer centers such as the Fred Hutchinson Cancer Research Center in Seattle use funds from private donations to pay scientists' salaries, for scientific equipment, and for testing new theories that may not yet be at a stage where they could get government funding. Breast cancer researchers and programs for women living with breast cancer need your financial help as well as your volunteer time. If you have only $5 to give, that goes a long way if a million women each join you giving $5! You can donate money to a cancer research center, a university that does cancer research, or local or national organizations that sponsor cancer research. You can also donate to local or national organizations that provide services to women who cannot afford to pay for breast cancer screening or treatment.

✍ Get Active

One of the best ways of showing support is by putting your interests into action. By getting physically active, you will not only get fitness benefits for yourself, you will also be a role model for other women and girls. The more women who are doing what they can to increase their exercise and their fitness, the more real will seem the demand by the government agencies that provide support for activities. For example, if you want your local community to build more bicycle paths, if you and your friends are out on your bikes frequently, and if you get other women to do the same, your community leaders will take your request for bike paths more seriously.

You can also be a role model for girls and young women. In too many of our schools, physical education classes are the first to be cut when the budgets are tight. Our young girls are getting driven to school since parents are concerned about their safety in walking to school. We now have a generation of girls who ride a school bus or are driven to school, sit all day in classes, and come home and flop on the couch to watch television or sit at the computer. If you are out exercising and participating in sports, you can influence the young girls in your community to get active as well.

Many communities around the country host noncompetitive fitness events including walks and runs that benefit breast cancer research, education, and treatment. You do not need to be an athlete to participate in these. You just have to be willing to walk a bit—you don't even have to finish the race. By participating, you help to fund breast cancer programs, you increase your fitness, and you inspire your more sedentary friends, relatives, and acquaintances to increase their fitness.

Summary

- All women and the men who support them must fight breast cancer. Scientists and clinicians are only one part of the team searching for prevention and cure. We need your help.
- Being a participant in a research study is an exciting and interesting way to contribute to the effort. Our study participants all bring a keen sense of adventure to our efforts.
- Local and national breast cancer organizations can use your help as a volunteer. You will gain much satisfaction in knowing that you are part of the larger world of women fighting against breast cancer.
- If you can donate money, consider donating to a cancer research center, a university, or an organization that sponsors cancer research or cancer programs.
- Be a role model. Get more physically active, and you'll not only benefit yourself, you'll also be an excellent influence on other women and on the children and teenage girls in your life and community.

Afterword

You are the master of your own body and your own destiny. If you are determined, you can make changes in your life that will benefit your health. Breast cancer is a formidable disease, but thousands of women around the world are fighting against the disease and are winning the battle.

Exercise and a healthy lifestyle are an important means to a critical end, that is, to improve your health and well-being. Whether you are a breast cancer survivor or are concerned about your risk for breast cancer, exercise can be a tool to reduce your risk and improve your quality of life.

We have given you a gift of our knowledge and experience. Your gift back to us will be to use the tools we have provided and put them into your everyday life. We derive great joy from seeing our patients, clients, and all women improve their lives through increasing exercise and making other beneficial lifestyle changes. We wish you well on your journey to a healthy and happy life!

Appendix A: Tools

How to Calculate Your Body Mass Index, or BMI

Your BMI is your weight corrected for your height. To calculate your BMI, you first need to convert your weight into kilograms and your height into meters. To calculate your weight in kilograms, divide your weight in pounds by 2.2. For example, if you weigh 145 pounds, you weigh 145 ÷ 2.2 = 65.9 kilograms. To calculate your height in meters, first calculate your height in inches. If you are 5 feet 2 inches, you are 12 x 5+2 = 62 inches tall. Multiply your height in inches by 2.5 and then divide by 100 to get your height in meters. If you are 62 inches tall, you are 62 x 2.5 ÷ 100 = 1.55 meters tall.

To calculate your BMI, now divide your weight in kilograms by your height in meters, then divide the number you get again by your height in meters. So if you weigh 65.9 kilograms and are 1.55 meters tall, your BMI is 65.9 ÷ 1.55 ÷ 1.55 = 27.4.

Doctors and obesity experts use the following ranges of BMI to determine whether a person is underweight, healthy weight, overweight, or obese.

Table A.1. Body Mass Index

BODY MASS INDEX	INTERPRETATION
Under 18.0	Underweight
18.0 –25.0	Healthy weight
25.1–29.9	Overweight
30.0 and above	Obese

You can also use computer programs that are available to calculate your BMI. There are free sites on the Internet that will calculate your BMI for you. Just search on body mass index using your favorite search engine.

✍ How to Measure Your Waist-to-Hip Ratio

You can determine your body shape by measuring your waist and your hip circumferences and then dividing your waist measure by your hip measure to get your waist-to-hip ratio. For example, if your waist is 30 inches and your hips are 40 inches, your waist-to-hip ratio is $30 \div 40 = .75$. If your waist-to-hip measure is .85 or greater, you have an "apple" shape.

Table A.2. Estimated Average Calories Burned per Hour for Women, by Weight

EXERCISE	110 POUNDS (50 KILOGRAMS)	130 POUNDS (59 KILOGRAMS)	150 POUNDS (68 KILOGRAMS)	170 POUNDS (85 KILOGRAMS)
IN-LINE SKATING	625	750	850	1050
KICK BOXING	500	600	675	850
RUNNING, 5.2 MPH	450	525	600	775
BACKPACKING	350	400	475	600
STATIONARY BIKE, 150 WATTS	350	400	475	600
SWIMMING LAPS	350	400	475	600
BASKETBALL	300	350	400	500
TENNIS, DOUBLES	300	350	400	500
BICYCLING, 10–12 MPH	300	350	400	500

EXERCISE	110 POUNDS (50 KILOGRAMS)	130 POUNDS (59 KILOGRAMS)	150 POUNDS (68 KILOGRAMS)	170 POUNDS (85 KILOGRAMS)
STAIR-CLIMBER	300	350	400	500
DANCE, AEROBIC, LOW IMPACT	250	300	350	425
WEEDING GARDEN	225	275	300	400
WALKING, 3.5 MPH	200	225	250	325
YOGA	200	225	250	325
WEIGHT LIFTING, MODERATE	150	175	200	250

You can calculate these numbers for yourself for your weight and for your specific activity. Just multiply your weight in kilograms (see above) by the met level for the specific activity (see below).

Table A.3. Met Levels of Various Exercises

ACTIVITY	MET LEVEL	ACTIVITY	MET LEVEL
In-line skating	12.5	Canoeing, rowing, moderate	7.0
Rowing, 200 watt	12.0	Soccer, general	7.0
Bicycling, 16–19 mph	12.0	Racquetball, general	7.0
Squash	12.0	Backpacking	7.0
Rock climbing, ascending	11.0	Walking, 4.5 mph	6.3
Stationary bike, 200 watt	10.5	Stair climber	6.0
Jumping rope, moderate	10.0	Weight lifting, vigorous	6.0
Judo, karate, kick boxing	10.0	Bicycling, 10–12 mph	6.0
Running, 6 mph	10.0	Mowing lawn, push mower	6.0
Running, 5.2 mph	9.0	Shoveling snow by hand	6.0
Rowing, 150 watt	8.5	Chopping wood	6.0
Carrying groceries upstairs	8.0	Downhill skiing, moderate	6.0
Cross country skiing, 4–5 mph	8.0	Tennis, doubles	6.0
Tennis, singles	8.0	Basketball, general	6.0
Running, 5 mph	8.0	Hiking, cross country	6.0
Aerobic dance, high impact	7.0	Walking, 3.5 mph uphill	6.0
Stationary bike, 150 watt	7.0	Aerobic dance, low impact	5.0
Ice skating, general	7.0	Cleaning gutters	5.0
Swimming laps, moderate	7.0	Snorkeling	5.0

ACTIVITY	MET LEVEL	ACTIVITY	MET LEVEL
Water skiing	7.0	Kayaking	5.0
Softball or baseball	5.0	Walking, 3 mph	3.3
Walking, 4 mph	5.0	Ballroom dance, slow	3.0
Badminton, social	4.5	Weight lifting, moderate	3.0
Weeding	4.5	Carpentry, general	3.0
Painting, indoor	4.5	Diving	3.0
Golf, walking	4.3	Volleyball, noncompetitive	3.0
Yoga	4.0	Walking, 2.5 mph	3.0
Raking leaves	4.0	Cooking	2.5
Treading water	4.0	Cleaning, light	2.5
Tai chi	4.0	Washing dishes	2.3
Horseback riding, general	4.0	Driving a car	2.0
Walking, 3.5 mph	3.8	Sexual activity, vigorous	1.5
Vacuuming	3.5	Standing	1.5
Golf, using power cart	3.5	Sitting	1.0

Source: Adapted from B. E. Ainsworth et al., "Compendium of Physical Activities: An Update of Activity Codes and MET Intensities." *Medicine in Sports and Exercise* (1999); and B. E. Ainsworth et al., "Compendium of Physical Activities: Classification of Energy Costs of Human Physical Activities." *Medicine and Science in Sports and Exercise* 25 (1992): 71–82.

Appendix B: Resources

 ## Recommended Reading

Anderson, Bob. *Stretching*. Berkeley, CA: Shelter Publications, 1990.

Baily, Covert. *The New Fit or Fat?* Boston: Houghton Mifflin, 1991.

Batmanghelidj, F., M.D. *Your Body's Many Cries for Water,* Falls Church, VA: Global Health Solutions, 1992.

Edwards, Sally. *Heart Rate Monitor Guide Book to Heart Zone Training.* Adelaide, Australia: Performance Matters, 1997.

———. *Heart Zone Training*. Adelaide, Australia: Adams Media Corp., 1996.

———. *Triathlons for Women*. Sacramento, CA: Heart Zones, 1992.

———. *The Heart Rate Monitor Book for Cyclists*. Boulder, CO: Velo Press, 2000.

Feldman, Andrew. *The Jock Doc's Repair Kit: The New Sports Medicine for Recovery and Increased Performance*. New York: St. Martin's Press, 1999.

Foldi, Michael, M.D., and Ethel Foldi, M.D. *Lymphedema: Methods of Treatment and Control*. Lymphedema Society of Victoria, Medicina Biologica, 1991.

Garrison, Robert, Jr., and Elizabeth Somer. *The Nutrition Desk Reference*. New Canaan, CT: Keats Publishing, 1995.

Keim, Rachel. *The Cancer Lifeline Cookbook: What to Eat Now*. Seattle: Sasquatch Books, 1996.

Love, Susan, M.D. *Dr. Susan Love's Breast Book*. Reading, MA: Addison-Wesley, 1990.

Melpomene Institute for Women's Health Research. *The Bodywise Women*. Champaign, IL: Human Kinetics, 1990.

Nelson, Miriam, M.D. *Strong Women Stay Slim*. New York: Bantam Doubleday Dell, 1998.

———. *Strong Women Stay Young*. New York: Bantam Doubleday Dell, 1997.

Stumm, Diana, P.T. *Recovering from Breast Surgery*. Alameda, CA: Hunter House, 1995.

Swirsky, Joan, R.N. *Coping with Lymphedema*. Wayne, NJ: Avery Publishing Group, 1998.

Video

Focus on Healing Through Movement and Dance: For the Breast-Cancer Survivor
The Lebed Method
(800) 366-6038

Organizations for Cancer, Exercise, and Health Information

National Organizations

American Cancer Society (ACS)
A nationwide toll-free hot line provides information on all forms of cancer and referrals to the American Cancer Society's "Reach to Recovery" program.
(800) ACS-2345
www.cancer.org
www.cancer.org/bcn/index.html (ACS breast cancer network)

FORCE: Facing Our Risk of Cancer Empowered
A Web site and chat room for women at increased risk for breast or ovarian cancer.
www.facingourrisk.org

The Susan G. Komen Breast Cancer Foundation
Sponsors annual Race for the Cure events in more than 100 cities across the country, which support breast cancer research, outreach, and treatment.

5005 LBJ Freeway, Suite 370
Dallas, TX 75244
(972) 855-1600
(800) IM-AWARE (toll-free hot line)
www.komen.org

National Action Plan on Breast Cancer
Established in 1994 as a partnership between the Department of Health and
   Human Services and the community to develop a plan to eradicate breast
   cancer. Web site has good information and links.
www.napbc.org

National Alliance of Breast Cancer Organizations (NABCO)
A nonprofit resource for information and education about breast cancer.
9 East 37 Street, 10th floor
New York, NY 10016
(888) 80-NABCO
www.nabco.org

National Association for Continence
Educational resources on incontinence, including treatment options and management. Audiotapes available for pelvic floor (Kegel) exercise and general
   pelvic health.
(800) BLADDER

National Breast Cancer Coalition
Active in obtaining increased funding for breast cancer research.
1707 L Street NW, Suite 1060
Washington, DC 20036
(202) 296-7477
www.natlbcc.org

National Coalition for Cancer Survivorship
Raises awareness of and deals with issues related to cancer survivorship.
1010 Wayne Avenue, Suite 770
Silver Spring, MD 20910
(877) 622-7937
www.cansearch.org

National Lymphedema Network
A nonprofit organization providing information and referrals to lymphedema
    patients.
Latham Square
1611 Telegraph Ave., Suite 1111
Oakland, CA 94612-2138
(800) 541-3259
www.lymphnet.org

The National Women's Health Information Center
A Web site on women's health managed by the Office on Women's Health of
    the Department of Health and Human Services.
www.4woman.org

Oncolink
A Web site from the University of Pennsylvania Cancer Center, with excellent
    cancer information and links to other Web sites.
oncolink.upenn.gov

Study of Tamoxifen and Raloxifene (STAR) Trial
National Surgical Adjuvant Breast and Bowel Project (NSABP)'s Web site
www.nsabp.pitt.edu

The Wellness Community National Offices (men and women)
Wellness centers. offering support groups, exercise and health classes, and
    resource center. Wellness centers throughout the country.
(888) 783-WELL
www.wellness-community.org

Women's Intervention Nutrition Study (WINS)
A study evaluating dietary fat in breast cancer survivors.
Call (800) 4-CANCER to see if there is a site near you.

Y-ME National Breast Cancer Organization
Provides breast cancer information and support. Offers trained peer counselors
    to callers of their toll-free hot line.
212 W. Van Buren Street
Chicago, IL 60607

www.y-me.org
(800) 221-2141
Spanish language: (800) 986-9505

The YWCA of the USA's Encore Plus Program
Located at YWCAs throughout the country. Provides breast cancer outreach
and exercise services to all women.
(800) 95-EPLUS

Gilda's Club Inc.
Offers support and networking groups, lectures, workshops, and social events
on emotional and physical well-being throughout the country.
(212) 647-9700
www.gildasclub.org

National Cancer Institute

Cancer Information Service (CIS) of the National Cancer Institute
The nation's education and information site on all aspects of cancer. Provides
informational brochures, refers callers to medical centers and clinical trials
programs.
(800) 4-CANCER (422-6237)
cancernet.nci.nih.gov

National Cancer Institute's Web site on prevention, early detection, and
genetic testing
Rex.nci.nih.gov/PREV_AND_ERLYDETC/PREVED_MAIN_DOC.html

National Cancer Institute's Clinical Trials Web site
Cancertrials.nci.nih.gov

National Cancer Institute RISK Computer Program
National Cancer Institute Cancer Information Service
(800) 4-CANCER (422-6237)
http://207.121.187.155/NCI_CANCER_TRIALS/zones/Forms/NciSignUp_
3.html

STAR Trial Information
National Cancer Institute Cancer Information Service

(800) 4-CANCER (422-6237)

http://cancertrials.nci.nih.gov/NCI_CANCER_TRIALS/zones/TrialInfo/
News/star/index.html

Author Affiliations

Fred Hutchinson Cancer Research Center

A national comprehensive cancer center.

The mission of the Fred Hutchinson Cancer Research Center is the elimination of cancer as a cause of human suffering and death. The center conducts research of the highest standards to improve prevention and treatment of cancer and related diseases.

1100 Fairview Avenue North

PO Box 19024

Seattle, WA 98109

(206) 667-5000

www.fhcrc.org

University of Washington Breast Cancer Specialty Center

1959 NE Pacific Street

Seattle, WA 98195

(206) 598-4104

www.washington.edu/medical/uwmc/uwmc_clinics/bcsc/index.htmI

Cancer Lifeline (men, women, and families)

Offers exercise and health-related classes as well as emotional support programs at their Dorothy O'Brien Center. Cancer Lifeline also provides a 24-hour help line, a Kids & Parents program, nutrition and cooking classes, and an extensive Arts and Healing program. Services and classes are open to all cancer patients and survivors as well as family and friends.

6522 Fremont Avenue N

Seattle, WA 98103

Program information: (206) 297-2100

24-hour Lifeline: (206) 297-2500

Toll-free (in Washington state): (800) 255-5505

www.cancerlifeline.org

Team Survivor Organizations (Women)

See Chapter 13 for detailed Team Survivor information.
www.teamsurvivor.org lists all programs and contact information

Team Survivor Northwest
200 NE Pacific Street, Suite #101
Seattle, WA 98105
(206) 732-8350
www.teamsurvivornw.org

Team Survivor–California
(310) 829-7849

Team Survivor–DFW
(972) 423-6282

Team Survivor–Austin, Breast Cancer Resource Center of Austin
(512) 472-1710

Rocky Mountain Team Survivor–Boulder, Colorado
(303) 247-1212

Appendix C: Sample Exercise Logs

S A M P L E

Weekly Exercise Log	Zone Name	% of Max. Heart Rate
	1. Redline	90–100%
	2. Threshold	80–90%
	3. Aerobic	70–80%
	4. Temperate	60–70%
	5. Healthy Heart	50–60%

Date	Sport/Exercise Activity	Distance	Time	Heart Rate Zone	Comments
S					
M					
T					
W					
TH					
F					
S					

S A M P L E

Weekly Exercise Log	Zone Name	% of Max. Heart Rate
	1. Redline	90–100%
	2. Threshold	80–90%
	3. Aerobic	70–80%
	4. Temperate	60–70%
	5. Healthy Heart	50–60%

Date	Sport/Exercise Activity	Distance	Time	Heart Rate Zone	Comments
S	Walk	2.8 miles	43 min	Zone 2	Greenlake, walked with Ellen, felt good
M	Walk	4.1 miles	55 min	Zone 1	Bridge walk, tired, long day at work
T	Walk		30 min	Zone 3 rainy-cold	Bridge walk (short),
W					Day off
TH	Walk	2.8 miles	45 min	Zone 2	Greenlake, walked with Ellen, good day!
F	Walk		60 min	Zone 2/3	Discovery Park, some hills, felt okay
S	Golf				16 holes with David—no cart

Glossary

benign breast disease. Growths and tumors in the breast that are not cancerous and are not dangerous to the woman.

body mass index (BMI). Weight corrected for height (see Appendix A for how to calculate your BMI).

breast biopsy. The removal of a small amount of breast tissue (glands and surrounding structures) so that it can be studied under a microscope to look for cancer. Biopsies can be done with a surgeon's knife or with a large hollow needle.

breast carcinoma in situ. An early stage of breast cancer, in which the tumor is still only in the breast where it first developed, and the disease has not invaded other parts of the breast or spread (metastasized). Most in situ carcinomas are highly curable.

breast cyst. A lump in the breast that is filled with fluid. It is almost always benign, although some can be cancerous. The fluid can be removed with a needle for analysis.

breast self-examination. A woman's regular (usually monthly) examination of her own breasts by visual inspection and palpation with her fingers.

cancer initiation. The first event that starts the cancer process. An initiated cell may or may not grow into a detectable tumor.

cancer promotion. The second and later event that cause an initiated cancer cell to grow without regulation into a collection of tumor cells.

carcinogen. Any substance that causes cancer or promotes its growth. Known or suspected breast carcinogens include excessive radiation and estrogen.

case-control study. An epidemiological study where data from persons with and without a disease are compared to look for factors that might be associated with the development of the disease.

chemotherapy. Drug treatment. Can be given by intravenous administration, injection, or by mouth.

clinical trial. A research study where individuals are assigned to one or more treatments by chance. The treatments can be pills, exercise programs, shots, diets, etc. Usually, some individuals are assigned by chance to a control group, for comparison with the treatment group. The control can be the standard treatment in the case of patients, or can be no treatment in the case of well individuals in a diet clinical trial.

cohort study. An epidemiological study where a number of individuals are identified at one time point, data are collected on them, and they are followed forward in time to identify who develops disease. The data in those who develop disease are compared with data from those who do not develop disease. The Women's Health Initiative has a cohort study of almost 94,000 women as one of its components.

epidemiology. The science of the causes and distribution of disease. Epidemiologists can be physicians or Ph.D.-trained scientists.

estrogen. A female sex hormone produced primarily by the ovaries in women who have not gone through menopause or had their ovaries removed. After menopause, the main source of estrogen in women is fat tissue. Estrogen regulates the development of breasts and other sexual organs, helps to regulate the monthly menstrual cycle, and helps to prepare the body for fertilization and reproduction. High levels of estrogen predispose a woman to develop breast cancer. In breast cancer patients, estrogen may promote the growth of cancer cells.

genes. The pieces of all cells' DNA that code for specific proteins. Several genes are involved in the process of cancer initiation, promotion, and control. There are genes that can kick-start a cancer, and genes that can shut down a cancer.

hormone. A chemical substance produced in your body, usually in a gland, that affects other parts of your body. The hormone travels through the bloodstream and sets in motion various body functions. Estrogen, testosterone, and insulin are examples of hormones. Prolactin, a hormone that is produced in the pituitary gland, begins and sustains the production of milk in the breast after childbirth.

hormone replacement therapy. Estrogen that is given to women whose ovaries no longer product estrogen. It is usually combined with proges-terone in women who still have a uterus.

hyperplasia. Abnormal cell growth. It is not cancer; not dangerous to the woman.

immune system. The parts of the body that interact to defend the body against invaders. The invaders can be from the outside, as with viruses or bacteria. The invaders can be cancer cells if the body sees them as being foreign.

invasive breast cancer. Cancer cells that have invaded surrounding normal tissue or elsewhere in the body.

lumpectomy. The surgical removal of a breast cancer lump without the removal of the entire breast.

lymph nodes. Small bean-shaped collections of immune system tissue such as lymphocytes, located along lymphatic vessels. They remove waste and fluids from lymph and help fight infections. Also called lymph glands.

lymphatic vessel. Vessels that carry lymph fluid, which transports infection-fighting substances and cells around the body.

lymphedema. Swelling in the arm caused by excess fluid that collects after lymph nodes and vessels are removed by surgery or treated by radiation. An infrequent complication after breast cancer treatment.

malignant. Cancerous, having the ability to grow and spread and destroy tis-sue; not benign.

mammogram. Low-dose X-ray examination of the breasts to look for breast cancer.

mastectomy. Surgical removal of the breast, either for breast cancer treat-ment or to prevent the development of breast cancer. Mastectomies have been done in rare cases for painful cystic breasts and for treatment of infec-tions or trauma.

menopause. The time in a woman's life when monthly cycles of menstruation cease forever and the level of hormones produced by the ovaries decreases. Menopause usually occurs in the late forties or early fifties, but it can also be caused by surgical removal of both ovaries (oophorectomy), or by some chemoptherapies that destroy ovarian function.

metastasis. The spread of cancer cells to distant areas of the body by way of the blood or lymphatic systems.

National Cancer Institute (NCI). The part of the National Institutes of Health that is devoted to cancer research. It pays for most of the cancer prevention studies done in this country.

oncologist. A doctor who specializes in the diagnosis and treatment of cancer.

percent body fat. The proportion of your body that is composed of fat tissues. For most women this should be between 20 and 28 percent.

progesterone. A female hormone that is involved in menstrual function and pregnancy. In hormone replacement therapy, it is usually given with estrogen to women who have a uterus.

proliferation. The biological process whereby one cell grows into several cells. Proliferation can be a normal body process if it occurs in the right cells and right part of your body. Proliferation can lead to cancer if it goes unchecked.

prophylactic mastectomy. Removal of breast tissue to prevent breast cancer. Sometimes the skin and nipple are left to preserve normal appearance. Other times, the nipple is removed and an artificial nipple is constructed.

protocol. The blueprint of a research study. The protocol lays out the rationale for doing the study, research design, the overall procedures, and the plans for evaluation of results.

tamoxifen. A therapy commonly used to treat breast cancer. It acts to block estrogen from promoting cancer growth in some tumors. It is now also approved for use in women without breast cancer, to reduce risk of breast cancer development. It is the first drug approved for this purpose.

Index

About the Authors

Anne McTiernan, M.D., Ph.D., is an international leader in research on exercise and other methods to prevent breast cancer occurrence and recurrence. She is a scientist at the Fred Hutchinson Cancer Research Center and research associate professor at the University of Washington. Her scientific findings have been published in the *New England Journal of Medicine* and other major scientific publications, magazines, and newspapers. She lives near Seattle, Washington.

Julie Gralow, M.D., is an assistant professor of medical oncology, specializing in breast cancer, at the University of Washington and the Fred Hutchinson Cancer Research Center. She is director of the University of Washington's Women's Cancer Genetics and Risk Reduction Clinic. She is co-chair of the Southwest Oncology Group's Breast Cancer Committee and serves as medical director for Team Survivor Northwest. She lives in Seattle, Washington.

Lisa Talbott has been teaching exercise to individuals and groups for over nineteen years. As a fitness and therapeutic exercise specialist, Lisa cofounded Team Survivor, a national nonprofit organization that teaches women cancer survivors how to use exercise for physical and emotional recovery. She is the health promotion manager at Cancer Lifeline and is completing her graduate studies in public health education. She lives in Seattle, Washington.